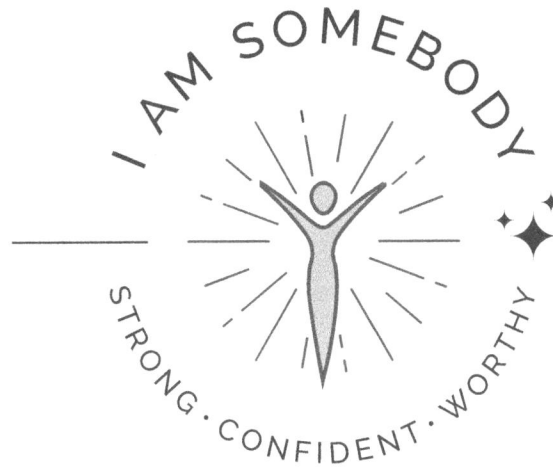

I AM SOMBODY

Transform Your Life Organizer™

Jennifer Bulbrook

I am Somebody
Transform Your Life Organizer
Jennifer Bulbrook

1st Edition. 1st printing 2021

Cover Concept Design and Interior Design: Steve Walters, Oxygen Publishing Inc.

Oxygen
PUBLISHING   AGENCY
AUTHORITY BY THE BOOK

Independently Published by
Oxygen Publishing Inc.
Montreal, QC, Canada
www.oxygenpublishing.com

ISBN: 978-1-990093-25-8
Imprint: Independently published

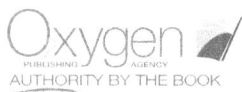

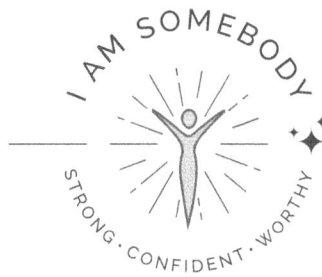

I AM SOMEBODY

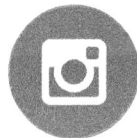

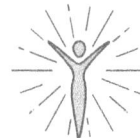

Mission Statement

I Am Somebody provides the highest quality of wellness while bringing strength and abundance to our clients by sharing personal experiences and incorporating new techniques into our daily lives!

I Am Somebody is dedicated to offering a unique experience through inspiration and motivation to everybody by showing them that they Are Somebody, no matter their mental health.

We own who we are because We Are Somebody!

Vision Statement

I Am Somebody provides a safe space to promote growth and encourage you to explore a deep sense of belonging.

I Am Somebody!
Strong! Confident! Worthy!

I Am Somebody!
Inspire! Empower! Honor! Promote! Encourage!

I Am Somebody!
Powerful! Strong! Control! Live!

I Am Somebody!

FIND JENNIFER ONLINE

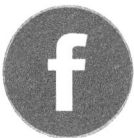

@IAM_SOMEBODY_2   @IAM_SOMEBODY_2   www.iamsomebody2.ca   coachId=2083073

Welcome to the beginning of your brand-new life.

The journey of a thousand miles begins with a simple step, and this, my friend, is your step.

Task: Make a commitment to yourself that from this day forward you are the only person you are setting out to please. I do not mean be selfish, I mean take notice your wants and needs, and use your voice.

Congratulations on purchasing this Self Coaching Planner, you are now on your way to not only getting organized and sticking with it but you will now experience a more balance life. Are you ready to not only believe in yourself and your dreams, but to say goodbye to your excuses and negative patterns? You ready to receive POSITIVE support throughout your journey as you are reminded… say it with me… **I Am Somebody.**

Well let me tell you, you have just taken the first step to organizing your life and allowing yourself to be Somebody. Allow yourself the life you have always wanted! We are always giving to others whether it is our time, our love, our energy and usually to the point where we forget about ourselves. Well, the time is NOW for you to start taking care of yourself. Focusing on ourselves is one of the most unselfish things we can do and why… Say it with me… I Am Somebody!

I am Jennifer Bulbrook, the Founder and Owner of the new Canadian Brand, I Am Somebody and I will be your person to help you to your brand-new life which is waiting for you within these pages. My hope is to be able to not only inspire you but to teach you the tools and skills you need to fulfill your dreams and to stand proud as you scream, **I Am Somebody!**

Our Transform Your Life Self Coaching Planners will feature self-development strategies, and each will be specifically geared towards topics such as Self-Worth, Addiction, Anxiety, Moving on from a relationship etc. A list of Self-Coaching Planner will be available to you at WWW.IAMSOMEBODY2.ca. These planners will also be available on Amazon.

What You Can Expect

Life Transformation

We will be working together to ensure you have the best life possible. I will be assisting you in your journey and supporting you in any way I can.

As I mentioned earlier, each Self Coaching Planner will be geared toward a certain topic such as Depression, Self-Worth, etc and because of this you may find different subtopics, information, worksheets and tasks in each.

Each month will begin with a topic such as Goal Setting, Self-Love, Decluttering, Buffering, etc. There will be a short write up for you to read followed by a worksheet.

The weekly spread includes little exercises/tasks which I strongly encourage you to complete. They are here to help you throughout your journey to give you the best experience possible. Some of these tasks will be written, where you may have some questions to answer. Some of these may be physical, where you may go for a walk, another may be mental where you may be asked to sit quietly and reflect on your day.

You can complete the written tasks under the Notes Sections throughout the book or in your thought download journal or buy a book just for this. Once you complete the task, you may take a picture or video of the done said task, post it on Facebook or Instagram, tag I Am Somebody and have your name entered for a draw @IAM_SOMEBOSY_2 #IAM_SOMEBODY_2.

On the daily spread you will find an am and a pm page with great self developmemt tools for you to implemenet into your daily lives. Each page also contains an area for your Thought Download, a space where you can unleash your mind.

Also, there is a podcast that coincides with each topic we discuss in these Self Coaching Planners and some, for example, there will be episodes on topics such as Goal Setting, Decluttering and Thought Download as well as many more. So as these topics in this Self Coaching Planner come up, click over, and have a listen to the podcasts. If this does not seem to be addressed in our podcast section of our website, please feel free to send in a suggestion. I am trying to cover everything and will be adding new content regularly. It is to your benefit to take advantage of not only the tasks but the podcasts to ensure you receive the most out of this journey.

I have designed this specific Self-Coaching Self-Worth Planner for anyone who is experiencing a low sense of esteem and/or worth, someone who is feeling as though they do not matter, or maybe you just feel as though something is missing but you are not sure what. I have gathered the tools that have helped me to feel alive and happy and am now offering them to you. The one thing we all as humans desire is to be happy. I know if you commit to yourself and to this Self Coaching Planner you will feel the world of a difference. I have also decided while designing these that I need to go further, I need to jump all in and really make sure that I am giving you the highest quality care possible, and I went ahead and enrolled myself at The Life Coach School where I studied under the amazing Brooke Castillo. I am incorporating what I am learning with each of these Transformation Self Coaching Planners to ensure great changes in each of you.

We are going to create a balance life, no matter where we are in our lives, we can be truly happy and I am excited to help show you the way. Throughout our journey we will be discussing what the true source of our happiness is and we will learn how to create it. You create our own feelings with what you think and therefore… just by changing your thoughts, you can find the true balance in your life.

As you are loving your amazing journey and thinking, you want even more then visit The Squad at www.iam_somebody_2.ca where we work closely one on one where we take all of this information and apply it in real time.

And Remember if you do not put the work in, the change will not happen.

You Got This

Say it with me…
I Am Somebody!!!

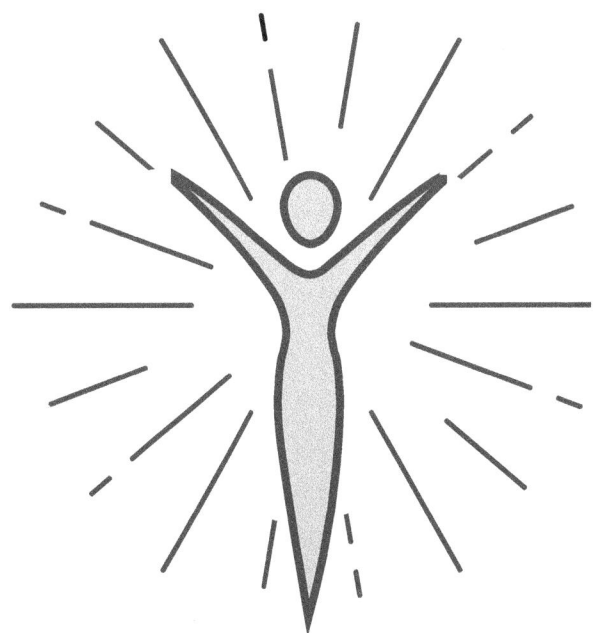

DREAM LIFE.

Believe in yourself and believe you can do anything you want in this life.

Since you have purchased this amazing *Transform Your Life Organizer™* I assume that you are ready to feel amazing and ready to not only believe in yourself and your dreams but to say goodbye to your excuses and negative patterns. You will receive POSITIVE support throughout your journey as you are reminded… say it with me… I Am Somebody.

If you have been feeling like you need a change, or something is missing but are just not sure what it is, here are some questions to help you decide what it is that you want in your life. Even if you came into this knowing what your goal is going to be, answer the following questions anyways, you may be surprised to what you find.

WHAT ARE SOME OF THE AMAZING THINGS THAT HAVE HAPPENED IN MY LIFE?

WHAT WOULD HAVE MADE THE LAST MONTH/SIX MONTHS BETTER?

WHAT WILL MAKE MY DAYS AHEAD GREAT?

WHAT MAKES ME HAPPY?

JENNIFER BULBROOK

DREAM LIFE.

From the answers you provided on the previous page,
it is now time to brainstorm goal ideas in the space provided below.

- _____
- _____
- _____
- _____
- _____
- _____
- _____
- _____
- _____
- _____
- _____
- _____
- _____
- _____

After you have come up with your ideas, I want you to go back and ask yourself which ones are going to serve you most? What ones will have the biggest positive impact on your life? Score them from 1 to 10 (10 being the one to serve you most) You may have the same score for more then one answer.

GOAL SETTING.

Work Smarter Not Harder

Do not rely on reaching your goals to make you happy. Don't think that once you reach your goal, that magically, happiness shows up. Unfortunately, it doesn't work that way because true happiness comes from within and in fact, the best time to make changes is when you are happy. You are going to find that as you navigate your journey, that by the time you accomplish your goals you set out to do, you are going to already be happy. You cannot expect outside factors to make you happy. Happiness comes from your thoughts so until you change the way you think, it will not matter what changes are made externally. I will be talking more about this throughout your journey.

To begin, we must decide on your 2 main goals which help you evolve and inspire to become better versions of yourself than you were yesterday. Look back at your responses from Dream Life and choose which goals you would like to work on and from there develop a clear specific vision by using the SMART approach. This will not only help you to accomplish your goals, but it will also allow you to feel and see your goals as you are working on them.

SPECIFIC- Be clear and detailed- What do we want to achieve and why? Who is involved? Where and when will this happen?

MEASURABLE- How will we know we have achieved our goal?

ATTAINABLE- Is the goal within reach and how can we meet our goal?

RELEVENT- Are the goals relevant to where we want to be or what we want to change?

TIMELY- Important to give time frame for our goals. As we plan each step and the amount of time to achieve each. It provides great motivation to have a deadline.

GOAL CATEGORY IDEAS– DREAM BIG yet have some balance

SELF- BODY, MENTAL HEALTH

JOB/CAREER/FINANCES

HOME LIFE

RELATIONSHIPS

LEISURE TIME/HOBBIES

Because our brain is always trying to protect us, you may notice that once you begin to make specific goals with specific plans and due dates, your brain will automatically begin to list all the reasons why your goals are not achievable or suited for you. Do not be discouraged or give up, this is normal and there is an actual technique which will help you overcome this hurdle.

Where are you now? Where do you want to be? What is going to stop you from getting there? As your brain begins the negative talk with respect to your goals, don't ignore it, but instead I want you to acknowledge and listen without judgment. Do NOT agree but hear it and write down all the negative talk and obstacles your mind is telling you which may sound like: "I don't know how to do this," "I have never done that before," "That will not work if..." etc....

Now that you have acknowledged your obstacles which are just your thoughts, it is time to change them into your strategies or mini goals. For instance, if your obstacle was "I am not tech savvy" then you can covert this into a goal where you learn tech things. Remember not to judge your thoughts as good or bad.

LET'S GOAL SET - What works for me

CATEGORY	6 MONTH GOALS
GOAL #1 **Mind & Body**	Be at my healthiest mentally including: Loving myself unconditionally To be able to feel excited about the next day To have control over my moods To be productive Be at my healthiest physically including: Toned all over - 6 pack abs - Nice booty Loose 12 pounds of fat Gain 12 pounds of muscle
GOAL #2 **Career**	Own my successful Brand I Am Somebody Website up & running - large amount of traffic Podcast up and running with thousand dedicated followers. Helping thousands of people through my various planners, designed around topics such as getting over ex, sobriety, self love etc.

IN ORDER TO ACHIEVE OUR 6 MONTH GOALS, WE MUST PLAN ON WHERE WE NEED TO BE IN 1 MONTH, 3 MONTHS AND 5 MONTHS.

6 MONTH GOAL	1 MONTH	3 MONTHS	5 MONTHS
GOAL #1 -Mind & Body Be at my healthiest mentally: Loving myself unconditionally. To feel excited about life. To be in control over my moods. Be productive Be at my healthiest physically. Toned - 6 pack abs - Nice booty Loose 12 pounds of fat Gain 12 pounds of muscle	Completed the Mind Over Mood Workbook Feeling good about myself- learning to accept my flaws Able to get up & out of bed most days Be down 3 pounds of fat Gained 3 pounds of muscle	Completed the first half of The Life Coach School Podcasts on YouTube Beginning to love myself and accept who I am Able to get out of bed and in decent mood most days Be down another 3 pounds of fat =6 Gained another 3 pounds of muscle = 6	Completed the second half of The Life Coach School Podcasts on YouTube Loving myself and where my life is going I look forward to getting out of bed and starting my day Be down another 3 pounds of fat =9 Gained another 3 pounds of muscle = 9
GOAL #2 -Career Own my successful Brand I Am Somebody Website up & running - large amount of traffic Podcast up and running with thousand dedicated followers. Helping thousands of people through my various planners and courses each specifically designed around topics such as getting over ex, sobriety, self love etc. Make $10,000	Logo and colours are chosen Apply for the Trademark online by February 30 Buy the podcast equipment by February 30 Complete my first 2 planners without podcast by March 30 Get Instagram and Facebook account for I Am Somebody by April 7 Reach out for any help at any time	Record podcasts for planners by June 30 4 Planners out for review and feedback from family & friends Begin to work on Website by July 30 Begin posting in social media sites Research and contact various printers Advertise Reach out for any help at any time	Planners are at printers by date printers suggest for launching Jan 2022 Have website up and running with podcasts and linked to all social media and other sites I may have Getting ready to Launch Advertise Reach out for help at any time

IN ORDER TO SUCCEED WITH OUR 1-, 3- AND 5-MONTH PLANS, WE MUST DETERMINE WHAT THE STEPS ARE TO GET THERE. What is best course of action? What changes need to happen? Resources?

6 MONTH GOAL	MONTHLY	WEEKLY	DAILY
GOAL #1 - My Mind & Body Be at my healthiest mentally including: Loving myself unconditionally To be able to feel excited about the next day and be productive instead of laying around all day and eating takeout regularly Body Be at my healthiest physically Toned all over - 6 pack abs - Nice booty Loose 12 pounds of fat Gain 12 pounds of muscle	Re-evaluate goals, needs and plan... change where needed Stick with my routines and re-evaluate when and where needed Self development practice including Podcast/Affirmatio/Reflections daily/Self development book Loose 1 pounds of fat Gain 1 pound of muscle High protein diet Less sugar More water Shakeology daily Workout 5/week Less sleep eating Healthy eating Do not lay in bed all day	Re-evaluate goals, needs and plan... change where needed Self development practice including Review Week. Podcast/Affirmatio/Reflections daily Self development book chapter each day stick to a morning and evening routine High protein intake Shakeology 5-6 days Workout 5-6/week less sleep eating Meal plan & preparation Do not buy junk	Self development practice including Podcast/Affirmatio/Reflections daily Self development book chapter each day stick to a morning and evening routine High protein diet healthy eating Drink Shakeology Workout sleep 7 hrs/night No more sleep eating Minimum sugar intake Alternate sugar cravings for Healthier options
GOAL #2- Career Own my successful Brand I Am Somebody Website up & running - large amount of traffic Podcast up and running with thousand dedicated followers. Helping thousands of people through my various planners and courses each specifically designed around topics such as getting over ex, sobriety, self love etc. Make $10,000	Review month. Re-evaluate goals, needs and plan... change where needed list accomplishments of the month list things that need to improve on Reach out for any help at any time Be All In No Excuses Be Confident Remember I Am Somebody	Review Week. Re-evaluate goals, needs and plan... change where needed Subtle hints on social media sites Work on planner 5 Mon to fri Research Reach out for any help at any time Be All In No Excuses Be Confident Remember I Am Somebody	Work on Planners – write up 3-5hrs/day Work on researching various things with respect to brand/podcast/website/planners 1-2hrs/day Reach out for help at any time Be All In No Excuses Be Confident Remember I Am Somebody

YOUR GOAL SET - LET'S DO THIS! ... WE GOT THIS!

"A Goal Without A Timeline Is Just A Dream" Robert Herjavec.
Its Time to Make Those Dreams into Our Reality

CATEGORY	6 MONTH GOALS

IN ORDER TO ACHIEVE OUR 6 MONTH GOALS,
WE MUST PLAN ON WHERE WE NEED TO BE IN 1 MONTH, 3 MONTHS AND 5 MONTHS.

6 MONTH GOAL	1 MONTH	3 MONTHS	5 MONTHS
GOAL #1			
GOAL #2			

JENNIFER BULBROOK

IN ORDER TO SUCCEED WITH OUR 1-, 3- AND 5-MONTH PLANS, WE MUST DETERMINE WHAT WE NEED TO DO TO GET THERE. What is best course of action? What changes need to happen? Resources?

6 MONTH GOAL	MONTHLY	WEEKLY	DAILY
GOAL #1			
GOAL #2			

LET'S DO THIS! ... WE GOT THIS!

FOCUS WORD

You get what you focus on, so focus on what you want and/or need

Now that you have identified your goals, it is time for you to choose a Focus Word or Statement that summarizes them up. I recommend answering these questions:

1. What do you need more of?

2. What do you want to focus on?

3. What do you feel you need to improve on?

4. WHY? Why do you need more of what you need? Why do you want to focus on what you do? Why do you feel you need to improve on what you want too? Why do you want this change?

Here are a few examples of focus words or statements that you can use:

I Am Somebody, Embrace, Free, Courage, Strength, Transform, Grace, Cultivate, Trust, Replenish, Grow, Believe, Heal, I am worthy, Committed, or Rejuvenate.

On page 16 you will, in a nutshell, brainstorm your chosen Focus Word vision board, as demonstrated on the next page. It will help give you emotion behind your chosen word or statement as well as encourage you to use it when making decisions in your daily lives.

VISION BOARD PLANNER - 6 MONTH DREAM - MY EXAMPLE

FOCUS WORD What is my focus word or statement and what does it mean to me?

I AM SOMEBODY

For so long, as far back as I can remember, I never felt as though I really mattered or that I was anybody, never mind anybody special. Well, its my time to not only feel but to BELIEVE that I do matter, and I am not just anybody, **I AM SOMEBODY**.

FEELINGS	**GOALS**	**THINGS**
How do I want to feel?	What do I want to achieve?	What material things do I need or want?
Happy	Self confidence	Microphone
Proud	A Brand that will help others	Headphones
Accomplished	Series of planners	Microphone arm
Loved	Close relationship with family	New desk
Respected	Podcast, website	Lukas SIN #
Confident	6 pack abs	Performance Line
Calm	At my healthiest mentally	Shakeology

YOUR BODY	**VALUES**	**MY BEST**
Are you healthy? Are you strong? Do you have a healthy relationship with food?	What is most important to me?	I am at my best when
Pretty healthy	Family	I am working out
Have muscle	Friends	I am using my planner
Thin	Myself	I am being busy
Chocolate is weakness	Being happy and content in life	I am being listened to
Vodka is weakness	Happy home	There is quiet
Bad knees in the room	Being successful	There is mutual respect
Bad lower back	Honesty, respect	_____

VISION BOARD PLANNER - 6 MONTH DREAM

FOCUS WORD What is my focus word or statement and what does it mean to me?

_____

_____

_____

_____

FEELINGS

How do I want to feel?

_____

_____

_____

_____

_____

_____

GOALS

What do I want to achieve?

_____

_____

_____

_____

_____

_____

THINGS

What material things do I need or want?

_____

_____

_____

_____

_____

YOUR BODY

Are you healthy? Are you strong? Do you have a healthy relationship with food?

_____

_____

_____

_____

_____

VALUES

What is most important to me?

_____

_____

_____

_____

_____

MY BEST

I am at my best when

_____

_____

_____

_____

_____

HOW TO DISPLAY YOUR VISION?

After completing the Vision Board Planner, you are now ready to put your vision on display by either creating a visual board with text and images or by writing a detailed description of the feelings, things, and experiences that you want in your life.

Creating a vision board is designed to attract your feelings and emotions while providing inspiration and motivation through visual images and texts. Please note setting up a vision board is only effective if you use it so make sure to display it somewhere you will see it often.

If you are anything like me and not so creative, then you might decide to go with drafting a detailed description. Again, it is only effective if you use it, so make sure you read it daily; once in the morning and once before bed. You will gain motivation along with a clear reminder of why you are working so hard.

You can also take a picture of your vision board whether you decided to do a visual arrangement or a written description and save it on your phone and refer to it when needed throughout your day.

Make sure that you believe in what you put on your vision board. You must believe that these things will happen, and your emotions must match your vision, or the change will not happen. BELIEVE IN YOURSELF.

One more thing: focus on the Why and the How will Show Up!

Wake up each morning with a fire inside of you for that vision you are about the create … why?… Because…Say it with me… *I Am Somebody!*

MY VISION - MY EXAMPLE

Create that beautiful AFTER STORY that you can start living NOW even if you're before story is miles away from where you wan to be." Tonya Leigh

Date: January 7, 2020 - I AM EVOLVING, I AM SOMEBODY

I am at my healthiest and happiest, physically, and mentally, feeling the best I have in as long as I can remember. I have my moods under control, without medication. I am no longer snapping on people but rather speaking in a calmy respectful manner. My depression and anxiety barely show themselves anymore and when they do, I can take control of both. I am communicating in a positive way and taking responsibility for my thoughts. I am still smoke free. I drink on occasion and with zero blackouts. I am drug and pill free. I am no longer sleep eating. My body is all toned including my 6-pack abs and toned butt. I feel amazing, I look amazing. **I Am Somebody**

I completed The Life Coach School and I'm on my way to become a successful life coach where I have many clients and followers. I have created my own Brand, I Am Somebody, which provides the highest quality of wellness while bringing strength and abundance to our clients by sharing personal experiences and incorporating new techniques into our daily lives! I Am Somebody is dedicated to offering a unique experience through inspiration and motivation to everybody by showing them that they Are Somebody, no matter their mental health status, ethnic background, career, personality, education, or wealth. We own who we are because We Are Somebody! Our Brand website receives high traffic where we feature self development strategies, sell several Transform Your Life Organizer™ books, each specifically geared towards topics such as self-worth, depression, sobriety, moving on from a relationship, anxiety, etc....I have a successful Podcast with over a million followers where we discuss serious issues, funny things, feelings, experiences, etc. I am in the process of writing a book. On top of all these amazing accomplishments, I have reached the top of our team with respect to Beachbody. I have made my money back plus my first $10,000 in my first six months of business and then doubled that the following 6 months. **I Am Somebody**

The kids and I are closer now, they respect me more then they ever have before. They help me around the house and without me even having to ask. We say good morning, good night, ask how our days have been, we hang out. It has been great, and we all are happy. I see my grandson a couple times a month and there is no blame game being played by any party. We are all building our relationships and has been positive experience. We all enjoy our time we spend together. **I Am Somebody**

My boyfriend and I get along so great. We barely argue and when we do, we can nip it in the bud before turning into an outburst. We have mad respect and love for one another. We cuddle every night and hold hands when walking. We are always touching one another, showing, and sharing our feelings. We are both getting our needs met and understand that it is on me to make me happy and on him to make him happy. We understand that he is here for me to love him and I am here just for him to love me, no strings attached. ***I AM SOMEBODY***

MY VISION

Time to make yourself a priority and create your vision, why?... Because...say it with me... *I Am Somebody!* (*Images and Texts and/or Detailed Description*)

OUR THOUGHTS CONTROL OUR OUTCOME

Our emotions must match our belief of reaching our goals

We have the power to make our lives amazing with a magical tool that we already own, our thoughts. Thoughts are sentences in our minds which are spontaneous yet usually have a pattern. From the moment we wake up our minds begin to think, begin to spit sentences at us automatically with usually little control from us.

In a recent study done in Canada by Queens University and according to Dr. Jordan Poppenk, an expert in the field of cognitive neuroscience, people think approximately 6,200 thoughts every day. The study consisted of subjects watching movies while identifying when one thought ends and one begins, which researchers have labelled as "thought worms". According to Poppenk, "Thought worms are adjacent points in a simplified representation of activity patterns in the brain. When a person moves onto a new thought, they create a new thought worm that we can detect. We also noticed that thought worms emerge right as new events do when people are watching movies. Drilling into this helped us validate the idea that the appearance of a new thought worm corresponds to a thought transition."

Our thoughts are what give us positive emotions such as happiness, gratitude, joy, and inspiration. Changing your thinking and practicing positivity over time will reshape your life and change how you view yourself. But did you know that 80% of our thoughts are found to be not just negative, but repetitive? Most people do not intentionally choose their thoughts, and because they are on a constant cycle, we are often left feeling bad and without really knowing why we are feeling so bummed. We have control over our thoughts and throughout our journey, we will be practicing ways to think intentionally so that we can break those patterns that we want to break.

Our thoughts create our feelings. Our feelings create our actions which create our results! BANG!! To reach your goals, you'll need to focus on your thoughts and allow your emotions to fuel your results ahead of time. Our emotions can act as a barrier from us reaching our results and it is up to us to tear down those barriers that our minds put up to grow and reach our full potential.

While I write this, while I plan each day with building this Brand, I have butterflies in my stomach, the little hairs on my arms are standing up, with a tingling feeling on the back of my neck. I can not only see but feel the accomplishments ahead. I can taste my growth and my potential. I can see all the success that I am going to have in helping millions of people, having a successful Podcast and my Transform Your Life Organizer™ being the #1 hit worldwide. I can not only see it, taste it, and feel it but I believe it. When I picture all this success, I am allowing my thoughts to fuel my inspiration, my motivation, my confidence and ultimately it will be what helps me reach my goals. I cannot help but want to work towards my dreams when I am already feeling this amazingness and it is only the beginning of this journey of mine.

IT IS TIME TO BELIEVE WE ARE SOMEBODY

Now that we have identified what changes are required and have briefly touched on how thoughts are the key to everything, NOW is the time to make your dream life into a reality. Having a vision and goal is great but if you don't act on them, it doesn't matter. If you plan your day or week, you will get more accomplished.

Schedule time to work on your goals and commit to spending this time working on what is important to you. No excuses, make time as you deserve it and why? say it after me... *I Am Somebody!*

Yes, I know there is a lot of hard work along the way and some may say is "bullshit" that lies between us and our goals. That's ok because that stuff is supposed to be there. This makes us stronger and prepares us for when we do reach our goals. So, when we are about to give up, we are going to remember that we are stronger than our challenges and those challenges we will embrace with open arms. We Got This!

DON'T FORGET - There will be a few exercises/tasks throughout the **Transform Your Life Organizer™** which I strongly encourage you to complete that will help you throughout your journey to give you the best experience possible. Once you complete the task, you may take a picture or video of the said task, post it on Facebook or Instagram, tag I Am Somebody and have your name entered for a draw.

We also have Podcasts that coincide with each topic. For example, there will be episodes on topics such as Goal Setting, Decluttering, Thought Downloads, and more. So as these topics come up, listen to the corresponding Podcast episode.

ENJOY THIS: Transform Your Life Organizer
AND REMEMBER YOU ARE WORTH IT!

YOU ARE SOMEBODY!

I BELIEVE IN YOU AND NOW IT IS TIME FOR YOU TO BELIEVE IN YOU!

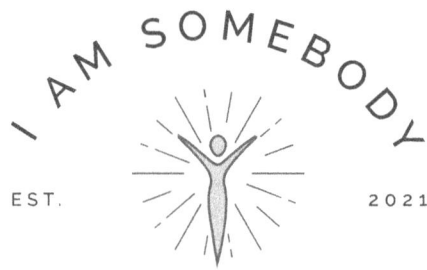

SAMPLE MONTH --- FEBRUARY

TIME TO CHECK IN:

My accomplishments Last month?

Lost 1 pound of fat.

Researched microphones and chose which one.

Kids and I went to Niagara Falls.

Worked on planner 6 days.

Areas I can do better next month? More or less of...

Stick with my workout routine.

Be more consistent on social media.

Take notes listening to podcast.

Research Trademark

MONTH AT A GLANCE - FEBRUARY

Use the space below space to write down any important upcoming events or deadlines you may **have** for the month.

NOTES	MONDAY	TUESDAY	WEDNESDAY
	5 Research Trademark	6 Report Due	7
	12	13 Sign up for Beachbody	14 Research and choose headphones to buy
	19	20 Phone bill due $255.00	21
	26	27	28

MONTHLY GOALS EXAMPLE

6 MONTH GOAL	MONTHLY GOAL
GOAL #1 – Mind & Body - Be at my healthiest mentally including: Loving myself unconditionally To be able to feel excited about the next day To have control over my moods · To be productive- Hour1 process 50/50 balance of emotions · Improve my physical health including: Toned all over - 6 pack abs - Nice booty Loose 12 pounds of fat · Gain 12 pounds of muscle	Self development practice including Podcast/Affirmatio/Reflections daily/ Self development book Loose 1 pound of fat Gain 1 pound of muscle Remember I Am Somebody
GOAL #2 – Career - Make $10,000 monthly Own my successful Brand I Am Somebody Website up & running - large amount of traffic Podcast up and running with thousand dedicated followers. Helping thousands of people through my planners and coaching each specifically designed around topics such as getting over ex, sobriety, self love etc	Choose logo and colours Apply for the Trademark online Buy the podcast equipment Work on planner Mon-Fri 3-5hrs/day Remember *I Am Somebody*

WE WILL NEVER FIND TIME, WE MUST MAKE TIME

EVERY SUNDAY, REVIEW AND RE-EVALUATE YOUR GOALS. IDENTIFY ANY OBSTACLES THAT YOU HAVE FACED ALONG WITH SOLUTIONS. .

THURSDAY	FRIDAY	SATURDAY	SUNDAY
1 Mom coming 9am for 4 days	2 Mom here	3 Mom here	4 Mom leaves tonight after dinner
8 Choose microphone and arm	9 Buy dumbbells Look into Web Designers	10	11
15 Zoom call with family @3pm	16 Colour scheme?? Logo??	17 Jessica and Max Here	18
22	23	24 Phone bill due $255.00	25

WE CAN DO ANYTHING WE PUT OUR MIND TO   Say it with me... **I AM SOMEBODY**

MY WEEK OF AWESOMENESS!
Now that our 6 month and monthly goals are done, we now can break down
our goals even further to make them even more achievable

REFLECTIONS OF LAST WEEK:

I only worked out 3 days

I ate out 2 days & struggled with sugar cravings almost every day.

I got great sleep all week and felt refreshed all week

Completed Self Development practice each morning as my routine

Chose I am going to begin my journey with I Am Somebody Brand

OBSTACLES I MAY FACE: Sugar cravings, special events with goodies and alcohol, money issues, name for Brand may not be available, self-doubt.

SOLUTIONS: Remind myself why I am doing this. Prepare healthy treats. Meal plan on Sundays. Drink Shakeology. Save money and do not spend recklessly. Remind myself I am worth it, *I Am Somebody.*

MY WEEK OF: FEBRUARY 5H TO 11TH

EACH WEEK YOU WILL BE GIVEN A TASK TO COMPLETE WHICH YOU WILL FIND HERE

TIME	MONDAY [5]	TUESDAY [6]	WEDNESDAY [7]
6am	Am Routine/ Energize	Am Routine/ Energize	Am Routine/ Energize
7am	Workout	Workout	Workout
8am	Drink Recover/Social	Drink Recover/Social	Drink Recover/Social
9am	Shower/Teeth	Shower/Teeth	Shower/Teeth
10am	Clean House		Clean House
11am	Mind Over Mood Book	Mind Over Mood Book	Mind Over Mood Book
12noon	Cheese Tray Kit	Grilled Tuna	Wieners and Beans
1pm	Work on Planner	Work on Planner	Work on Planner
2pm	Apply for Business License		
3pm			
4pm		Report due by 4pm	
5pm			
6pm	Ham Mash Corn	Steak Baked Squash	Chicken Rice C. Salad
7pm	Cuddle Time	Cuddle Time	Family movie Night
8pm	Phone Goes Away	Phone Goes Away	Phone Goes Away
9pm	Evening Routine	Evening Routine	Evening Routine
10pm	Bedtime	Bedtime	Bedtime
11pm			

MY WEEK OF AWESOMENESS!

6 Month Goal- Mind & Body	6 Month Goal- Career
Loose 12 pounds of fat	Own my own brand
Gain 12 pounds of muscle	
	MONTH- Logo & colours.
MONTH- Self-development practice including Podcast, Affirmation, Reflections etc	Apply for Business License. Research Trademark. Work on planner,
Loose 1 pound of fat.	
Gain 1 pound of muscle	**WEEK**- Finish 1 planner. Apply for business license.
WEEK- Self-development practice as morning routine	
Loose .5-pound fat.	**REWARD WHEN I REACH:**
Gain .25-pound muscle	Finish 1 hour early from work
REWARD WHEN I REACH:	
Put $10 toward new workout	

MY WEEK OF: FEBRUARY 5H TO 11TH

What time do you want to wake up at, go to bed? How do you want your week to look like?
What events or meetings do you need to attend? Are you planning on having a day of shopping?

THURSDAY [8]	FRIDAY [9]	SATURDAY [10]	SUNDAY [11]
Am Routine/ Energize	Am Routine/ Energize		
Workout	Workout	Am Routine/ Energize	
Drink Recover/Social	Drink Recover/Social	Workout	Am Routine
Shower/Teeth	Shower/Teeth	Drink Recover/Social	Groceries
Microphone and arm?	Web Designers	Shower/Teeth	
Mind Over Mood Book	Mind Over Mood Book	Clean & Laundry	
Chicken C. Salad	Toasted Egg	Grilled Tuna	Veggie Wrap
Work on Planner	Work on Planner	Work on Planner	Meal Plan
		Jessica and Max Here	
Zoom Call with Family			Family Boardgame
Spaghetti Garlic Toast	Sausage on bun fries	Date Night – Try Last Call Bar & Grill	Bacon Eggs Toast
Cuddle Time	Cuddle Time		Cuddle Time
Phone Goes Away	Phone Goes Away		Phone Goes Away
Evening Routine	Evening Routine		Evening Routine
Bedtime	Bedtime		Bedtime

AFFIRMATION OF THE DAY: I LOVE MYSELF ENOUGH TO PUSH THROUGH

TODAY, I AM LOOKING FORWARD TO
1. Seeing my grandson
2. Applying for my Master Business License
3. Having ham dinner.

GOALS #1 MIND & BODY	GOALS #2 CAREER	HABITS I AM TRACKING	Y/N
Workout	Draft intro of my first planner	Good morning Post	
Drink Performance Line	Apply for Master Business	Read Vision	
Drink Shakeology	License	Affirmation of The Day	
Drink Lots of Water	Futuristic	Excitement for Day	
Keep to Meal/Snack Schedule		Daily Goals	
8 Hours Sleep		Workout	
Complete 1 Chapter		Mind Over Mood Chapter	
Mind Over Mood		Listen to Podcast	
Listen to Podcast		Plans for Tomorrow	
Positive Affirmations		Phone Away	
Excitement for the Day			

THOUGHT DOWNLOAD

TODAY I AM CHOOSING TO FEEL:

C - Life, Mind & Body, Relationships, Business.

T - I have so many awesome things happening today.

F - Excited.

A - Show up, communicate, engage, follow my schedule, drink my shake and water, workout, visit with grandson, play like a kid at the park, think of future, tell everyone and anyone who will listen.

R - Had a great day filled with lots of excitement.

I WILL DRINK ___ GLASSES OF WATER TODAY: 1 2 3 4 5 6 7 8 9 10

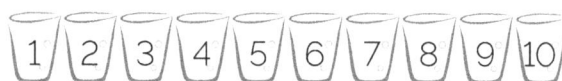

LOOKING BACK ON MY AMAZINGNESS

MY WINS I CELEBRATE TODAY ARE	TOMORROW I WILL IMPROVE ON
I stuck to my morning routine. I stuck to my meal plan. I calmed myself down after a negative comment from Chris and was able to let it go.	Having less self doubt and worry whether I will be successful.

3 THINGS I AM THANKFUL FOR LAST 24 HOURS:

1. Luka's mattress arrived
2. Chris cooked dinner
3. I completed more then I expected

THOUGHT DOWNLOAD

Overall feeling great today.

Had an argument with my boyfriend this morning because I was speaking, and he turned the volume up on his phone. I took it to believe he did not love me or care to hear what I was saying. I became incredibly angry and there was some yelling. ANGRY 100 & HURT 100
After thinking about it and completing the model, I realized that believing he did not love me or care about what I say was extreme. I then asked him why he turned the volume up. He stated he thought we were finished talking because there was silence and I had gone back to cleaning.

Circumstance- I was talking, bf was on the phone, bf turned volume on phone up.
Thoughts - he does not care, he is not listening, he does not even love me.
Feelings - angry, sad, hurt, frustrated.
Actions - yelling, banging things, snapping on bf.
Results –lose respect for one another, relationship suffers.

NOTES

The way to prevent these feelings, actions and results is to change the way we think. I could have asked him why or I could have decided to think that since I had paused that he assumed I was finished talking.

THE MORNING ROUTINE

I love the smell of possibilities in the morning.

I have never been a morning person. I already dreaded getting up and would press snooze about 20 times before getting my cranky miserable butt out of bed. The next few hours would consist of me trying to plan my day as I scrolled through Facebook. Throughout the day I was just miserable, controlling and just anxious and on edge all the time. Once I began my daily self- development practice, all of that changed. Now I wake up at 6am and send out a positive good morning post. I then spend 20-30 minutes listening to a podcast before reading my vision and completing my positive routine. My days are happier, calmer and a hell of a lot less anxious and my sleep has improved.

Mornings are difficult for most people but a morning ritual helps set the tone for the day and to better allow us to control our schedules rather than have our schedules control us. They say that the first hour of our day determines our next 23. Why not start it off right?

As we begin each day, an important question to ask is "why do we wake up?" What motivates us to do what we have planned for that day?

Knowing and understanding our "why" will strengthen our decision to wake up every day, prioritize our time and better focus on whatever challenges that may arise.

After reading my vision I find it beneficial to continue with positive talk as outline below:

Today I am looking forward to… Name 3 things you are looking forward to each day	Future View of Myself/My Life… What do you want your future to look like? Where do you want to be?
Daily Goals Choose at least 2 daily goals	Affirmations Positive statement about oneself. I Am…

Make sure your morning routine excites and motivates you as
it will in doubt shape the remainder of your day.

MY EXAMPLE

WAKE UP TIME: 6am

Time

Time	
6am	Up and Make Wake Bed
	Good Morning Post
	Listen to Podcast/Read Vision - Drink Energize
	Affirmations/Excitement/Daily Goals
7am	Workout
8am	Power Hour/Drink Recover
9am	Shower/Teeth

THE EVENING ROUTINE

Set the Tone for The Next Day!

A positive evening routine is just as important as a morning one! It helps prepare us for the next day, and for a good well-rested night sleep and overall minimizes our resistance to getting what we need to do done.

I used to be right on the ball with my morning routine and my attitude and disposition showed just that during the day. What I found, however, was that as the evening hit, my attitude would change, I was not as pleasant. I realised that I was giving such great energy to my morning routine yet nothing to my evening and it was showing and more importantly I was feeling it. I found my mind was becoming tired, I was reverting to my old habits, being snappy, unpleasant, eating junk.

I would stay awake late having a difficult time settling in and falling asleep. My sleep would consist of me tossing and turning, having my TV on with my mind going crazy and then to boot, my restless body syndrome would kick in. I just could not fall asleep and when I did, I was up every half hour eating and usually something chocolate and/or smoking. It was horrible, I needed to plan to keep my mind alert and focused, and find another way to be committed to my progress. That is when I began practicing my evening routine. Now I am asleep by 10pm, I sleep through the night, no more sleep eating and when I wake up in the morning, I am feeling refreshed and ready for the day.

Taking just a few moments at the end of the day to reflect and celebrate your wins puts things into proper perspective and gives us encouragement for the coming day.

It is easy to take your day to bed, making it difficult to fall asleep. Clearing your head before sleep allows you to put aside the challenges of the day and ready your mind to shut down. There are numerous ways to do this which you will be participating in some throughout your journey, including 30 minutes prior to going to bed. You can switch it up each night if you like or do the same thing, it is completely up to you and what you are more comfortable with:

- Do a Thought Download
- Draw
- Meditation
- Light reading

Make sure your evening routine is calming and peaceful.

MY EXAMPLE

WAKE UP TIME: 6am

Time

Time	
6pm	Dinner
7pm	Wins/Plans/Thankful/Reflection/Improve Upon
	Wash Face/Teeth
8pm - 9pm	Cuddle Time/Watch TV or movie/PHONE AWAY
9.30pm - 10pm	Power Hour/Drink Recover
10pm	Bedtime

SLEEP: Invest in blackout curtains. I advise you only to put them down when you are going to sleep During the day, make sure you have a lot of sunlight coming in.

TIPS ON HOW TO MAKE YOUR DAYS RUN MORE SMOOTHLY

1. Schedule your Non-negotiables on your calendar first. Your work, self-development practices, meal prep, and workouts. Include your meal planning and clean up times! Treat them as an appointment with an important client.

2. Set a time limit for social media and email. Many of us spend our time scrolling through social media sites that next thing we know, the day is half over, and we have accomplished a whole lot of nothing.

3. Choose three main tasks per day on your calendar. If you complete these and nothing else, give yourself zero guilt. If you can do more, great. If you do less, do not judge yourself, repeat the process again the next day and begin with what you missed today.

4. Set aside concrete time for the family. It could be a school pick up, after you or your spouse are home or after you are both finished work. No phones, no work, just being present with one another.

These four things will help you be less stressed and more productive each day!

So many of us focus on what is not going well and what we are doing wrong. Although it is good to touch base with these things, don't focus on them.

Today, we will begin to focus on what is going well and what we are proud of. It does not matter how small; it just matters that you are proud.

I AM SOMEBODY!

_____
Your Name

Let's begin with a simple exercise. Check off the boxes that remind you of why You Are Somebody! If you do not happen to think the statement applies to you, jot the reason down beside *it*.

o I am incredible	o I am accepting
o I am loved	o I am beautiful
o I am a hard worker	o am respectful to others
o I am smart	o I am enough
o I am strong	o I am stronger than I was yesterday
o I am loving	o I am worthy
o I am fierce	o I am wanted
o I am courageous	o I am powerful
o I am amazing	o am capable of great things
o I am thoughtful	o I Am Somebody

Developing self-worth and confidence is a huge deal. Things like love, acceptance, encouragement, honesty, and appreciation are all beautiful things which you should be giving to yourself each day. While completing this journey you will find proof of all the ways you are amazing and- say it with me…
I Am Somebody!

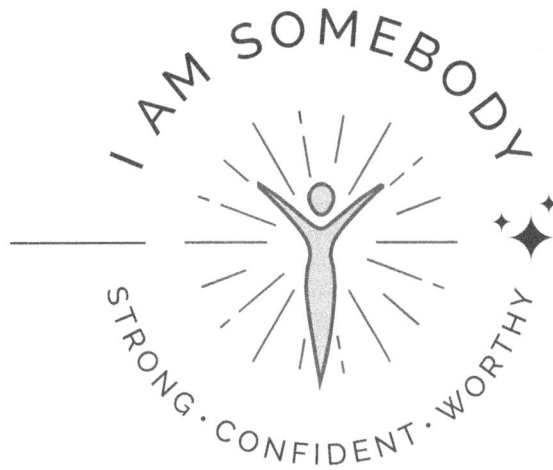

I AM SOMBODY

Transform Your Life Organizer™

Month One

DECLUTTER

It is possible to change these habits and to learn to let go, but you must make the time for it.

Imagine, piles of clothes and shoes in every room. Stacks of papers, books and bills covering countertops, possibly even the floors throughout your house. Storage spaces crammed with a little bit of everything.

What I just described to you is called clutter, and most people are not aware that clutter:

- Creates mental chaos.

- Is what we hold on to when we fear we do not have enough.

- Prevents productivity and growth.

- Can prevent you from achieving goals, dreams, aspirations.

- Causes stress.

- Plays a part in procrastination and vice versa.

- Causes a distraction.

- Can provide a sense of overwhelm.

Every six months I recommend you remove anything that you do not use regularly or anything that you have in multiples. Drop the excuses and get your habits on point. Since this **Transform Your Life Organizer™** is six months long, I recommend that you plan to complete your decluttering process at the same time as beginning your Organizer. It is perfect timing, really!

Do not feel guilty over keeping things over the other or not keeping this or that. These material items do not make you who you are, but they do influence one's mindset if you allow it. my dad passed away 16 years ago, and I ended up with his desk, which at the time I absolutely loved and would not have had it any other way. As the years went on, the desk began to wear and tear, and eventually began to fall apart. I began to not really like the desk, and became frustrated and annoyed with it. I know, it is just a desk. I just could not part with it though, no matter how many times I swore at it for the drawer handle falling off or the inside just falling apart, I just could not get rid of my dad's desk. I would complain about it to my mom, and she would say, your dad did not even really like that desk, but to me I just could not replace it. I could not even tell you how many times I went online or in a store and looked at the desks, but I could never buy one. Well guess what my friends, I finally replaced my dad's desk with a new one and well I absolutely love it and am so happy I chose not to let a desk have power over me. I will not allow myself to feel guilty for what is best for me, for what I want. Truth be told if my dad were alive, that desk would have been thrown out years ago and would not have waited this long and that is when I knew it was ok with me to get rid of it.

A great way to start decluttering is to throw away items that are:

- Broken
- Ruined
- No longer able to be used
- Normal trash items: old wrappers, lists, etc.

Ask yourself, would you buy it now? If yes, keep it.

If you were to move to a new place, would you bring it? If yes, keep it.

TASK: Take 1-5 days this month to go through all your belongings and what you do not use regularly or have multiple of them is time to part with them. When parting with anything that is not actual trash, donate or sell these items.

For each room, go in and complete the following task...

STEP 1- YOU'VE GOT THIS	STEP 2- SORT & TOSS
Take everything out of your cupboards, pantry, and closets depending on what room you are in. Clean the inside of the cupboards etc., whether wiping down the shelves with Lysol wipes or sweeping and mopping the closet floor. Yes, there will be big piles of your things now and it may look or feel overwhelming to you but just remember, Breathe, you are in control of your thoughts and you have the power to make this into a fun relaxing experience.	Go through everything you have taken out of your drawers, etc. and make categories such as garbage, closet, donate etc. Where needed, check the expiration date and throw away old items Toss anything you do not use or need. Remember the methods I had mentioned previously about would I buy it today? Etc. If it is something that can be sold or donated, please do that before just throwing it in the garbage. There are many people out there that can not afford to pay the price of new things or even old things.
STEP 3- THE FINISH LINE IS NEAR	STEP 4 – CONGRATULATIONS!
Wipe down all items that are not going into the garbage Label anything you need, whether it is items you have or the place you are going to put them. You can label them by name, date owned by etc. Place them in the proper place, make a home for all your things whether it be a drawer, donation box, garbage bag, closet etc	Take some time to reflect on all the hard work you just put into decluttering your beautiful home. Open a window, let the fresh air in, breathe, take pictures of your success. Take this as a freeing moment in your life. Next, we will be learning the importance of decluttering our minds!

LET'S DISCUSS OUR BELIEFS!

Our mind is the most powerful tool that allows us to have the things in life that we believe are possible. Our brains, our thoughts are the key to everything as what we believe is based on what we think over and over. Unfortunately, if we allow our thoughts of fear and doubt to take over, then our beliefs can have a negative effect.

Below I want you to write your thoughts that you have that you feel hinder your progress. Do NOT judge your thoughts!

Now ask yourself what evidence you have that supports these beliefs or thoughts? If I were to ask your friends or family, would they agree with these statements? Are you ready to change your beliefs? Remember we control what we think and ultimately believe, and we can believe whatever we want. What do you want to BELIEVE ABOUT YOU? What you believe is YOUR TRUTH!

Below, rewrite your beliefs by replacing them with positive statements that encourage your progress and shows support and confidence toward yourself. What new thoughts do you want to think to replace the ones that have been hindering and getting in the way?

Be realistic, as you must believe your thoughts. You cannot go from hating your body to loving your body, it is a gradual process so you can say that you are learning to love your body, or "I love my arms", etc.

Please note this is not a magical overnight skill; it can take days, weeks, or months to get to the positive belief. Come back to this list any time you need a reminder of how amazing and strong you are.

JENNIFER BULBROOK

DECLUTTERING YOUR MIND

Writing down your ideas, thoughts, feelings, tasks is smart not only because it gets them out of your head, creates mental space but gives you clarity on things in your life. This is one of the situations where your Thought Download Journal will help your progress. It is great to have all your thoughts in one tidy, organized space rather than notes everywhere. You want to avoid transferring the problem into creating physical clutter.

When you choose to declutter your minds, just like your home, it creates space in which you can gain perspective about your needs, the decisions you are making, goals, what needs to be changed and how to go about making those changes etc.

So many times, we have silly nonsense in our mind taking up a lot of space better spent acting upon your dreams and aspirations. If your mind is overflowing with thoughts of everything others are doing and worrying about outside of your control, then how do you expect not to feel overwhelmed when something new enters your life. How do you expect to fit new situations, experiences, and people into your life if you do not make room for them? Just like that junk drawer you just cleaned out; I'll bet before you tackled that drawer there was little room for anything else and now that it is complete, you have room for a nice sized book. It is great to replace those old thoughts with new motivating thoughts.

Decluttering does not have to be a stressful experience; whether it's your home, office, mind, or life. Relax, take a deep breath - this will not take up too much of your time, and we'll work little by little. Decluttering can be a freeing experience in which you embrace and feel such ease and happiness as a result.

We will begin small with a simple question which I want you to write in your Thought Download Journal or any type of notebook you have. Once you write the question, take the next 5-20 minutes writing about it. Keep on writing until the time is up or until there is nothing left in your thoughts, whichever one comes first.

First question: What are you going to get out of using this Transform Your Life Organizer™?

Just a few minutes of decluttering your mind sends a clear message that your life is becoming more spacious, organized, and manageable. Decluttering your mind does not only involves decluttering your environment and Thought Download Journals but many other exercises that you can do. You will continue to help with the clutter in your mind and life by using this *Transform Your Life Organizer™* along with the daily routines. Please follow the exercises as well.

If there are any decisions that you have been putting off, now is the time to take action on those decisions. Too many times our brains are indecisive on what it is we want or need and it takes up mad space in our minds.

Let go of any negative thoughts about your past that you have been holding onto that no longer serve you such as grudges or mistakes made, or heartbreak.

Face any problems you may have. I am not saying that you must confront everyone and all situations you have issues with, but you can use your Thought Download Journal to let out what's on your mind about the situation and/or person. Write non-stop until you feel there is nothing left to say. Sometimes this is all we need and when we do this, we feel clarity. At times we may even be ready to confront the person or situation head on.

THOUGHT DOWNLOAD JOURNAL

(Visit http://www.IAMSOMEBODY2.ca for our selection of Thought Download Journals)

WHAT YOU WILL NEED- pen/Thought Download Journal or notebook/or some sort of paper/10min- just write.

Sometimes you must find your thoughts—anxious, overwhelm to clean up the clutter in your mind

GREAT SOURCE TO FIGURE OUT ANYTHING YOU ARE DEALING WITH! You will learn to trust yourself, increase your self-confidence, learn more about your wants and needs, and to prove to yourself that say it with me... *I AM SOMEBODY!*

CAN'T SLEEP? Get out your pen and journal and start writing. Keep on writing until you feel like you have written everything on your mind

FEELING WORRIED? Some questions you may want to ask yourself are: What are you worried about? What scares you? What do you wish was different? What are you struggling with? What is your problem?

CAN'T FIGURE OUT WHY YOU ACTED A CERTAIN WAY? Write how you feel? What do you think? Keep writing, write nonstop for 10 minutes and you will see how your thinking is causing your results.

TASK: Decluttering your mind or house – which was easier for you? Why?

How did you feel after the de-clutter? After completing your first download. If I completed more downloads, which I would imagine you have, do you see a difference in you? Feeling less anxious, more at ease, less stressed? Better knowledge of oneself?

MONTHLY GOALS

START STRONG! YOU GOT THIS! I BELIEVE IN YOU NOW ITS TIME FOR YOU TO BELIEVE IN YOU!

"Stay true to yourself. An original is worth more than a copy" Suzy Kassem

6 MONTHS GOAL	MONTHLY GOAL
GOAL #1	
GOAL #2	

MONTH AT A GLANCE -

Take this space to write down any important upcoming events or deadlines you may have for the month.

NOTES			

WE WILL NEVER FIND TIME, WE MUST MAKE TIME

Every Sunday review & re-evaluate your goals. Identify obstacles that you faced, along with solutions.

		WE CAN DO ANYTHING WE PUT OUR MIND TOO	Say it with me… I AM SOMEBODY

MY WEEK OF AWESOMENESS!
Now that 6 month and monthly goals are done, we now can break down
our goals even further to make them even more achievable

REFLECTIONS OF LAST WEEK:

OBSTACLES I MAY FACE: _____

_____

SOLUTIONS: _____

_____

MY WEEK OF_____
Take 1-5 days this month to go through all your belongings and what you do not use regularly or have multiple of
them is time to part with them. When parting with anything that is not actual trash, donate or sell these items.

TIME			

MY WEEK OF AWESOMENESS!

6 Month Goal	6 Month Goal
MONTH	MONTH
WEEK	WEEK
REWARD WHEN I REACH	REWARD WHEN I REACH

MY WEEK OF_____

What time do you want to wake up at, go to bed? How do you want your week to look like?
What events or meetings do you need to attend? Are you planning on having a day of shopping?

AFFIRMATION OF THE DAY: _____

TODAY, I AM LOOKING FORWARD TO

GOALS #1	GOALS #2	HABITS I AM TRACKING	Y/N

THOUGHT DOWNLOAD

TODAY I AM CHOOSING TO FEEL:

C -

T -

F -
A -

R -

I WILL DRINK _____ GLASSES OF WATER TODAY: 1 2 3 4 5 6 7 8 9 10

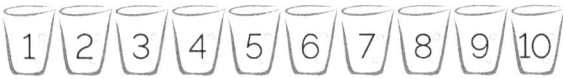

JENNIFER BULBROOK

LOOKING BACK ON MY AMAZINGNESS

MY WINS I CELEBRATE TODAY ARE	TOMORROW I WILL IMPROVE ON

3 THINGS I AM THANKFUL FOR LAST 24 HOURS:

1. ______________________________

2. ______________________________

3. ______________________________

THOUGHT DOWNLOAD

NOTES

AFFIRMATION OF THE DAY: _____

TODAY, I AM LOOKING FORWARD TO

GOALS #1	GOALS #2	HABITS I AM TRACKING	Y/N

THOUGHT DOWNLOAD

TODAY I AM CHOOSING TO FEEL:

C -

T -

F -
A -

R -

I WILL DRINK ___ GLASSES OF WATER TODAY: 1 2 3 4 5 6 7 8 9 10

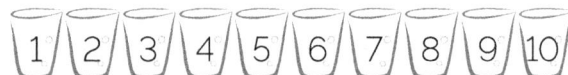

LOOKING BACK ON MY AMAZINGNESS

MY WINS I CELEBRATE TODAY ARE	TOMORROW I WILL IMPROVE ON

3 THINGS I AM THANKFUL FOR LAST 24 HOURS:

1. ______________________________

2. ______________________________

3. ______________________________

THOUGHT DOWNLOAD

NOTES

AFFIRMATION OF THE DAY: _____

TODAY, I AM LOOKING FORWARD TO

GOALS #1	GOALS #2	HABITS I AM TRACKING	Y/N

THOUGHT DOWNLOAD

TODAY I AM CHOOSING TO FEEL:

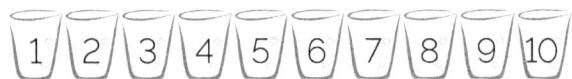

C -

T -

F -
A -

R -

I WILL DRINK ___ GLASSES OF WATER TODAY: 1 2 3 4 5 6 7 8 9 10

LOOKING BACK ON MY AMAZINGNESS

MY WINS I CELEBRATE TODAY ARE	TOMORROW I WILL IMPROVE ON

3 THINGS I AM THANKFUL FOR LAST 24 HOURS:

1. ______________________________

2. ______________________________

3. ______________________________

THOUGHT DOWNLOAD

NOTES

AFFIRMATION OF THE DAY: _____

TODAY, I AM LOOKING FORWARD TO

GOALS #1	GOALS #2	HABITS I AM TRACKING	Y/N

THOUGHT DOWNLOAD

TODAY I AM CHOOSING TO FEEL:

C -

T -

F -
A -

R -

I WILL DRINK ___ GLASSES OF WATER TODAY: 1 2 3 4 5 6 7 8 9 10

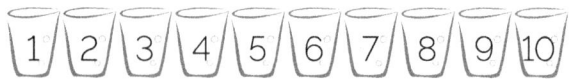

LOOKING BACK ON MY AMAZINGNESS

MY WINS I CELEBRATE TODAY ARE	TOMORROW I WILL IMPROVE ON

3 THINGS I AM THANKFUL FOR LAST 24 HOURS:

1. ______________________________

2. ______________________________

3. ______________________________

THOUGHT DOWNLOAD

NOTES

AFFIRMATION OF THE DAY: _____

TODAY, I AM LOOKING FORWARD TO

GOALS #1	GOALS #2	HABITS I AM TRACKING	Y/N

THOUGHT DOWNLOAD

TODAY I AM CHOOSING TO FEEL:

C -

T -

F -
A -

R -

I WILL DRINK ___ GLASSES OF WATER TODAY: 1 2 3 4 5 6 7 8 9 10

LOOKING BACK ON MY AMAZINGNESS

MY WINS I CELEBRATE TODAY ARE	TOMORROW I WILL IMPROVE ON

3 THINGS I AM THANKFUL FOR LAST 24 HOURS:

1. _____

2. _____

3. _____

THOUGHT DOWNLOAD

NOTES

AFFIRMATION OF THE DAY: _____

TODAY, I AM LOOKING FORWARD TO

GOALS #1	GOALS #2	HABITS I AM TRACKING	Y/N

THOUGHT DOWNLOAD

TODAY I AM CHOOSING TO FEEL:

C -

T -

F -
A -

R -

I WILL DRINK ___ GLASSES OF WATER TODAY: 1 2 3 4 5 6 7 8 9 10

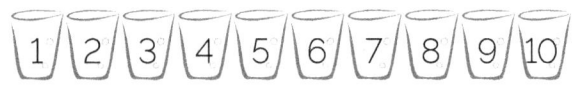

LOOKING BACK ON MY AMAZINGNESS

MY WINS I CELEBRATE TODAY ARE	TOMORROW I WILL IMPROVE ON

3 THINGS I AM THANKFUL FOR LAST 24 HOURS:

1. ______________________________

2. ______________________________

3. ______________________________

THOUGHT DOWNLOAD

NOTES

AFFIRMATION OF THE DAY: _____

TODAY, I AM LOOKING FORWARD TO

GOALS #1	GOALS #2	HABITS I AM TRACKING	Y/N

THOUGHT DOWNLOAD

TODAY I AM CHOOSING TO FEEL:

C -

T -

F -
A -

R -

I WILL DRINK ____ GLASSES OF WATER TODAY: 1 2 3 4 5 6 7 8 9 10

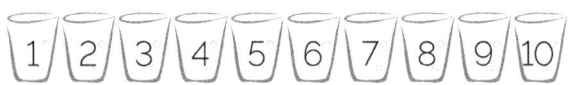

MY WINS I CELEBRATE TODAY ARE	TOMORROW I WILL IMPROVE ON

3 THINGS I AM THANKFUL FOR LAST 24 HOURS:

1. _____

2. _____

3. _____

THOUGHT DOWNLOAD

NOTES

MY WEEK OF AWESOMENESS!
Now that 6 month and monthly goals are done, we now can break down
our goals even further to make them even more achievable

REFLECTIONS OF LAST WEEK:

OBSTACLES I MAY FACE: _____

_____

SOLUTIONS: _____

_____

MY WEEK OF_____
Take 1-5 days this month to go through all your belongings and what you do not use regularly or have multiple of
them is time to part with them. When parting with anything that is not actual trash, donate or sell these items.

TIME			

MY WEEK OF AWESOMENESS!

6 Month Goal	6 Month Goal
MONTH	MONTH
WEEK	WEEK
REWARD WHEN I REACH	REWARD WHEN I REACH

MY WEEK OF_____

What time do you want to wake up at, go to bed? How do you want your week to look like?

What events or meetings do you need to attend? Are you planning on having a day of shopping?

AFFIRMATION OF THE DAY: _____

TODAY, I AM LOOKING FORWARD TO

GOALS #1	GOALS #2	HABITS I AM TRACKING	Y/N

THOUGHT DOWNLOAD

TODAY I AM CHOOSING TO FEEL:

C -

T -

F -
A -

R -

I WILL DRINK ___ GLASSES OF WATER TODAY: 1 2 3 4 5 6 7 8 9 10

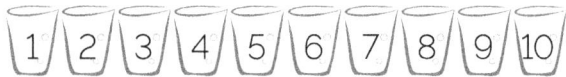

LOOKING BACK ON MY AMAZINGNESS

MY WINS I CELEBRATE TODAY ARE	TOMORROW I WILL IMPROVE ON

3 THINGS I AM THANKFUL FOR LAST 24 HOURS:

1. ______________________________

2. ______________________________

3. ______________________________

THOUGHT DOWNLOAD

NOTES

AFFIRMATION OF THE DAY: _____

TODAY, I AM LOOKING FORWARD TO

GOALS #1	GOALS #2	HABITS I AM TRACKING	Y/N

THOUGHT DOWNLOAD

TODAY I AM CHOOSING TO FEEL:

C -

T -

F -
A -

R -

I WILL DRINK ___ GLASSES OF WATER TODAY: 1 2 3 4 5 6 7 8 9 10

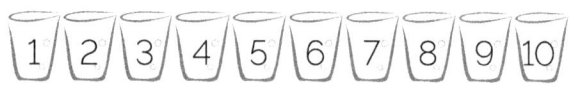

LOOKING BACK ON MY AMAZINGNESS

MY WINS I CELEBRATE TODAY ARE   TOMORROW I WILL IMPROVE ON

3 THINGS I AM THANKFUL FOR LAST 24 HOURS:

1. _____

2. _____

3. _____

THOUGHT DOWNLOAD

NOTES

AFFIRMATION OF THE DAY: _____

TODAY, I AM LOOKING FORWARD TO

GOALS #1	GOALS #2	HABITS I AM TRACKING	Y/N

THOUGHT DOWNLOAD

TODAY I AM CHOOSING TO FEEL:

C -

T -

F -
A -

R -

I WILL DRINK ___ GLASSES OF WATER TODAY: 1 2 3 4 5 6 7 8 9 10

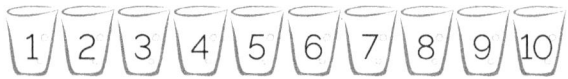

LOOKING BACK ON MY AMAZINGNESS

MY WINS I CELEBRATE TODAY ARE	TOMORROW I WILL IMPROVE ON

3 THINGS I AM THANKFUL FOR LAST 24 HOURS:

1. ______________________________

2. ______________________________

3. ______________________________

THOUGHT DOWNLOAD

NOTES

AFFIRMATION OF THE DAY: _____

TODAY, I AM LOOKING FORWARD TO

GOALS #1	GOALS #2	HABITS I AM TRACKING	Y/N

THOUGHT DOWNLOAD

TODAY I AM CHOOSING TO FEEL:

C -

T -

F -
A -

R -

I WILL DRINK ___ GLASSES OF WATER TODAY: 1 2 3 4 5 6 7 8 9 10

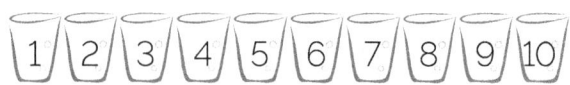

JENNIFER BULBROOK

LOOKING BACK ON MY AMAZINGNESS

MY WINS I CELEBRATE TODAY ARE	TOMORROW I WILL IMPROVE ON

3 THINGS I AM THANKFUL FOR LAST 24 HOURS:

1. ______________________________

2. ______________________________

3. ______________________________

THOUGHT DOWNLOAD

NOTES

AFFIRMATION OF THE DAY: _____

TODAY, I AM LOOKING FORWARD TO

GOALS #1	GOALS #2	HABITS I AM TRACKING	Y/N

THOUGHT DOWNLOAD

TODAY I AM CHOOSING TO FEEL:

C -

T -

F -
A -

R -

I WILL DRINK ___ GLASSES OF WATER TODAY: 1 2 3 4 5 6 7 8 9 10

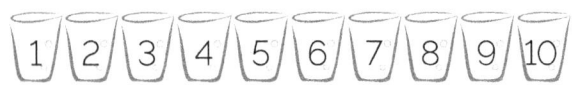

LOOKING BACK ON MY AMAZINGNESS

MY WINS I CELEBRATE TODAY ARE	TOMORROW I WILL IMPROVE ON

3 THINGS I AM THANKFUL FOR LAST 24 HOURS:

1. ______________________________

2. ______________________________

3. ______________________________

THOUGHT DOWNLOAD

NOTES

AFFIRMATION OF THE DAY: _____

TODAY, I AM LOOKING FORWARD TO

GOALS #1	GOALS #2	HABITS I AM TRACKING	Y/N

THOUGHT DOWNLOAD

TODAY I AM CHOOSING TO FEEL:

C -

T -

F -
A -

R -

I WILL DRINK ___ GLASSES OF WATER TODAY: 1 2 3 4 5 6 7 8 9 10

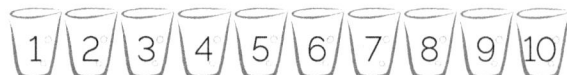

LOOKING BACK ON MY AMAZINGNESS

MY WINS I CELEBRATE TODAY ARE	TOMORROW I WILL IMPROVE ON

3 THINGS I AM THANKFUL FOR LAST 24 HOURS:

1. ______________________________
2. ______________________________
3. ______________________________

THOUGHT DOWNLOAD

NOTES

AFFIRMATION OF THE DAY: _

TODAY, I AM LOOKING FORWARD TO

GOALS #1	GOALS #2	HABITS I AM TRACKING	Y/N

THOUGHT DOWNLOAD

TODAY I AM CHOOSING TO FEEL:

C -

T -

F -
A -

R -

I WILL DRINK ___ GLASSES OF WATER TODAY: 1 2 3 4 5 6 7 8 9 10

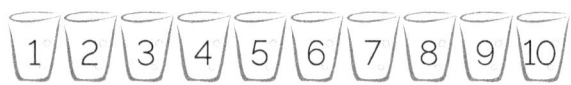

MY WINS I CELEBRATE TODAY ARE	TOMORROW I WILL IMPROVE ON

3 THINGS I AM THANKFUL FOR LAST 24 HOURS:

1. _____

2. _____

3. _____

THOUGHT DOWNLOAD

NOTES

MY WEEK OF AWESOMENESS!
Now that 6 month and monthly goals are done, we now can break down
our goals even further to make them even more achievable

REFLECTIONS OF LAST WEEK:

OBSTACLES I MAY FACE: _____

_____

SOLUTIONS: _____

_____

MY WEEK OF_____
Take 1-5 days this month to go through all your belongings and what you do not use regularly or have multiple of them is time to part with them. When parting with anything that is not actual trash, donate or sell these items.

TIME			

MY WEEK OF AWESOMENESS!

6 Month Goal	6 Month Goal
MONTH	MONTH
WEEK	WEEK
REWARD WHEN I REACH	REWARD WHEN I REACH

MY WEEK OF_____

What time do you want to wake up at, go to bed? How do you want your week to look like?
What events or meetings do you need to attend? Are you planning on having a day of shopping?

AFFIRMATION OF THE DAY: _____

TODAY, I AM LOOKING FORWARD TO

GOALS #1	GOALS #2

HABITS I AM TRACKING	Y/N

THOUGHT DOWNLOAD

TODAY I AM CHOOSING TO FEEL:

C -

T -

F -
A -

R -

I WILL DRINK ___ GLASSES OF WATER TODAY: 1 2 3 4 5 6 7 8 9 10

LOOKING BACK ON MY AMAZINGNESS

MY WINS I CELEBRATE TODAY ARE	TOMORROW I WILL IMPROVE ON

3 THINGS I AM THANKFUL FOR LAST 24 HOURS:

1. ______________________________

2. ______________________________

3. ______________________________

THOUGHT DOWNLOAD

NOTES

AFFIRMATION OF THE DAY: _____

TODAY, I AM LOOKING FORWARD TO

GOALS #1	GOALS #2	HABITS I AM TRACKING	Y/N

THOUGHT DOWNLOAD

TODAY I AM CHOOSING TO FEEL:

C -

T -

F -
A -

R -

I WILL DRINK ___ GLASSES OF WATER TODAY: 1 2 3 4 5 6 7 8 9 10

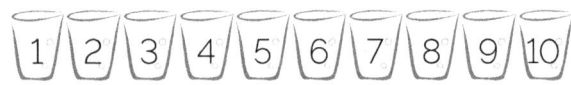

LOOKING BACK ON MY AMAZINGNESS

MY WINS I CELEBRATE TODAY ARE	TOMORROW I WILL IMPROVE ON

3 THINGS I AM THANKFUL FOR LAST 24 HOURS:

1. ______________________________
2. ______________________________
3. ______________________________

THOUGHT DOWNLOAD

NOTES

AFFIRMATION OF THE DAY: _____

TODAY, I AM LOOKING FORWARD TO

GOALS #1	GOALS #2	HABITS I AM TRACKING	Y/N

THOUGHT DOWNLOAD

TODAY I AM CHOOSING TO FEEL:

C -

T -

F -
A -

R -

I WILL DRINK ____ GLASSES OF WATER TODAY: 1 2 3 4 5 6 7 8 9 10

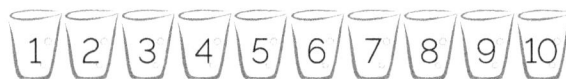

LOOKING BACK ON MY AMAZINGNESS

MY WINS I CELEBRATE TODAY ARE	TOMORROW I WILL IMPROVE ON

3 THINGS I AM THANKFUL FOR LAST 24 HOURS:

1. ______________________________

2. ______________________________

3. ______________________________

THOUGHT DOWNLOAD

NOTES

AFFIRMATION OF THE DAY: _____

TODAY, I AM LOOKING FORWARD TO

GOALS #1	GOALS #2	HABITS I AM TRACKING	Y/N

THOUGHT DOWNLOAD

TODAY I AM CHOOSING TO FEEL:

C -

T -

F -
A -

R -

I WILL DRINK ___ GLASSES OF WATER TODAY: 1 2 3 4 5 6 7 8 9 10

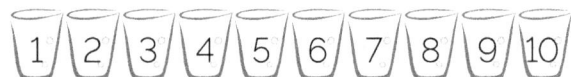

LOOKING BACK ON MY AMAZINGNESS

MY WINS I CELEBRATE TODAY ARE	TOMORROW I WILL IMPROVE ON

3 THINGS I AM THANKFUL FOR LAST 24 HOURS:

1. _____

2. _____

3. _____

THOUGHT DOWNLOAD

NOTES

AFFIRMATION OF THE DAY: _____

TODAY, I AM LOOKING FORWARD TO

GOALS #1	GOALS #2	HABITS I AM TRACKING	Y/N

THOUGHT DOWNLOAD

TODAY I AM CHOOSING TO FEEL:

C -

T -

F -

A -

R -

I WILL DRINK ___ GLASSES OF WATER TODAY: 1 2 3 4 5 6 7 8 9 10

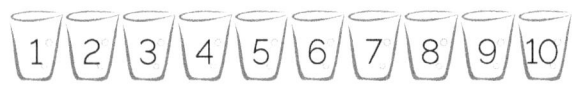

LOOKING BACK ON MY AMAZINGNESS

MY WINS I CELEBRATE TODAY ARE	TOMORROW I WILL IMPROVE ON

3 THINGS I AM THANKFUL FOR LAST 24 HOURS:

1. ______________________________

2. ______________________________

3. ______________________________

THOUGHT DOWNLOAD

NOTES

AFFIRMATION OF THE DAY: _____

TODAY, I AM LOOKING FORWARD TO

GOALS #1	GOALS #2	HABITS I AM TRACKING	Y/N

THOUGHT DOWNLOAD

TODAY I AM CHOOSING TO FEEL:

C -

T -

F -
A -

R -

I WILL DRINK ___ GLASSES OF WATER TODAY: 1 2 3 4 5 6 7 8 9 10

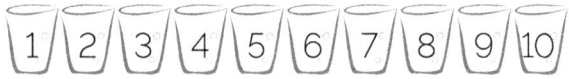

LOOKING BACK ON MY AMAZINGNESS

MY WINS I CELEBRATE TODAY ARE	TOMORROW I WILL IMPROVE ON

3 THINGS I AM THANKFUL FOR LAST 24 HOURS:

1. ______________________________

2. ______________________________

3. ______________________________

THOUGHT DOWNLOAD

NOTES

AFFIRMATION OF THE DAY: _____

TODAY, I AM LOOKING FORWARD TO

GOALS #1	GOALS #2	HABITS I AM TRACKING	Y/N

THOUGHT DOWNLOAD

TODAY I AM CHOOSING TO FEEL:

C -

T -

F -
A -

R -

I WILL DRINK ___ GLASSES OF WATER TODAY: 1 2 3 4 5 6 7 8 9 10

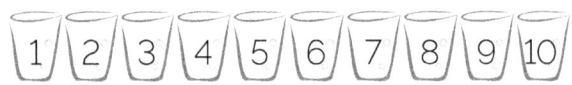

MY WINS I CELEBRATE TODAY ARE	TOMORROW I WILL IMPROVE ON

3 THINGS I AM THANKFUL FOR LAST 24 HOURS:

1. _____

2. _____

3. _____

THOUGHT DOWNLOAD

NOTES

MY WEEK OF AWESOMENESS!
Now that 6 month and monthly goals are done, we now can break down
our goals even further to make them even more achievable

REFLECTIONS OF LAST WEEK:

OBSTACLES I MAY FACE: _____

_____

SOLUTIONS: _____

_____

MY WEEK OF_____
Take 1-5 days this month to go through all your belongings and what you do not use regularly or have multiple of them is time to part with them. When parting with anything that is not actual trash, donate or sell these items.

TIME			

MY WEEK OF AWESOMENESS!

6 Month Goal	6 Month Goal
MONTH	MONTH
WEEK	WEEK
REWARD WHEN REACH	REWARD WHEN REACH

MY WEEK OF _____

What time do you want to wake up at, go to bed? How do you want your week to look like?
What events or meetings do you need to attend? Are you planning on having a day of shopping?

AFFIRMATION OF THE DAY: _____

TODAY, I AM LOOKING FORWARD TO

GOALS #1	GOALS #2	HABITS I AM TRACKING	Y/N

THOUGHT DOWNLOAD

TODAY I AM CHOOSING TO FEEL:

C -

T -

F -
A -

R -

I WILL DRINK ____ GLASSES OF WATER TODAY: 1 2 3 4 5 6 7 8 9 10

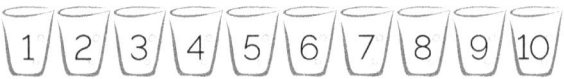

LOOKING BACK ON MY AMAZINGNESS

MY WINS I CELEBRATE TODAY ARE	TOMORROW I WILL IMPROVE ON

3 THINGS I AM THANKFUL FOR LAST 24 HOURS:

1. ______________________________

2. ______________________________

3. ______________________________

THOUGHT DOWNLOAD

NOTES

AFFIRMATION OF THE DAY: _____

TODAY, I AM LOOKING FORWARD TO

GOALS #1	GOALS #2	HABITS I AM TRACKING	Y/N

THOUGHT DOWNLOAD

TODAY I AM CHOOSING TO FEEL:

C -

T -

F -
A -

R -

I WILL DRINK ___ GLASSES OF WATER TODAY: 1 2 3 4 5 6 7 8 9 10

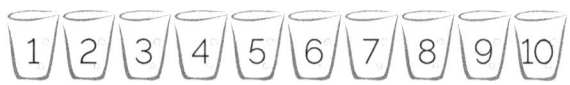

LOOKING BACK ON MY AMAZINGNESS

MY WINS I CELEBRATE TODAY ARE	TOMORROW I WILL IMPROVE ON

3 THINGS I AM THANKFUL FOR LAST 24 HOURS:

1. ______________________________

2. ______________________________

3. ______________________________

THOUGHT DOWNLOAD

NOTES

AFFIRMATION OF THE DAY: _

TODAY, I AM LOOKING FORWARD TO

GOALS #1	GOALS #2	HABITS I AM TRACKING	Y/N

THOUGHT DOWNLOAD

TODAY I AM CHOOSING TO FEEL:

C -

T -

F -
A -

R -

I WILL DRINK ___ GLASSES OF WATER TODAY: 1 2 3 4 5 6 7 8 9 10

JENNIFER BULBROOK

LOOKING BACK ON MY AMAZINGNESS

MY WINS I CELEBRATE TODAY ARE	TOMORROW I WILL IMPROVE ON

3 THINGS I AM THANKFUL FOR LAST 24 HOURS:

1. ______________________________

2. ______________________________

3. ______________________________

THOUGHT DOWNLOAD

NOTES

AFFIRMATION OF THE DAY: _____

TODAY, I AM LOOKING FORWARD TO

GOALS #1	GOALS #2	HABITS I AM TRACKING	Y/N

THOUGHT DOWNLOAD

TODAY I AM CHOOSING TO FEEL:

C -

T -

F -
A -

R -

I WILL DRINK ___ GLASSES OF WATER TODAY: 1 2 3 4 5 6 7 8 9 10

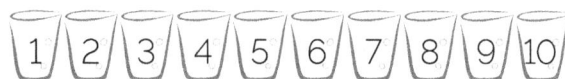

LOOKING BACK ON MY AMAZINGNESS

MY WINS I CELEBRATE TODAY ARE	TOMORROW I WILL IMPROVE ON

3 THINGS I AM THANKFUL FOR LAST 24 HOURS:

1. ______________________________

2. ______________________________

3. ______________________________

THOUGHT DOWNLOAD

NOTES

AFFIRMATION OF THE DAY: _____

TODAY, I AM LOOKING FORWARD TO

GOALS #1	GOALS #2	HABITS I AM TRACKING	Y/N

THOUGHT DOWNLOAD

TODAY I AM CHOOSING TO FEEL:

C -

T -

F -
A -

R -

I WILL DRINK ___ GLASSES OF WATER TODAY: 1 2 3 4 5 6 7 8 9 10

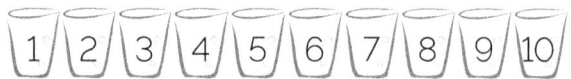

LOOKING BACK ON MY AMAZINGNESS

MY WINS I CELEBRATE TODAY ARE	TOMORROW I WILL IMPROVE ON

3 THINGS I AM THANKFUL FOR LAST 24 HOURS:

1. ______________________________

2. ______________________________

3. ______________________________

THOUGHT DOWNLOAD

NOTES

AFFIRMATION OF THE DAY: --

TODAY, I AM LOOKING FORWARD TO

GOALS #1	GOALS #2	HABITS I AM TRACKING	Y/N

THOUGHT DOWNLOAD

TODAY I AM CHOOSING TO FEEL:

C -

T -

F -
A -

R -

I WILL DRINK ___ GLASSES OF WATER TODAY: 1 2 3 4 5 6 7 8 9 10

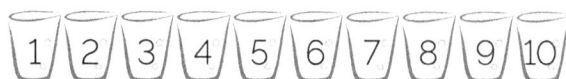

LOOKING BACK ON MY AMAZINGNESS

MY WINS I CELEBRATE TODAY ARE	TOMORROW I WILL IMPROVE ON

3 THINGS I AM THANKFUL FOR LAST 24 HOURS:

1. ____

2. ____

3. ____

THOUGHT DOWNLOAD

NOTES

AFFIRMATION OF THE DAY: _____

TODAY, I AM LOOKING FORWARD TO

GOALS #1	GOALS #2	HABITS I AM TRACKING	Y/N

THOUGHT DOWNLOAD

TODAY I AM CHOOSING TO FEEL:

C -

T -

F -
A -

R -

I WILL DRINK ____ GLASSES OF WATER TODAY: 1 2 3 4 5 6 7 8 9 10

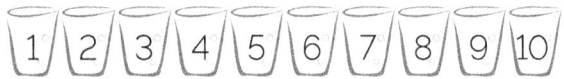

MY WINS I CELEBRATE TODAY ARE	TOMORROW I WILL IMPROVE ON

3 THINGS I AM THANKFUL FOR LAST 24 HOURS:

1. _____

2. _____

3. _____

THOUGHT DOWNLOAD

NOTES

MY WEEK OF AWESOMENESS!
Now that 6 month and monthly goals are done, we now can break down
our goals even further to make them even more achievable

REFLECTIONS OF LAST WEEK:

OBSTACLES I MAY FACE: _____

_____

SOLUTIONS: _____

_____

MY WEEK OF_____
Take 1-5 days this month to go through all your belongings and what you do not use regularly or have multiple of them is time to part with them. When parting with anything that is not actual trash, donate or sell these items.

TIME			

MY WEEK OF AWESOMENESS!

6 Month Goal	6 Month Goal
MONTH	MONTH
WEEK	WEEK
REWARD WHEN I REACH	REWARD WHEN I REACH

MY WEEK OF_____

What time do you want to wake up at, go to bed? How do you want your week to look like?

What events or meetings do you need to attend? Are you planning on having a day of shopping?

AFFIRMATION OF THE DAY: _

TODAY, I AM LOOKING FORWARD TO

GOALS #1	GOALS #2	HABITS I AM TRACKING	Y/N

THOUGHT DOWNLOAD

TODAY I AM CHOOSING TO FEEL:

C -

T -

F -
A -

R -

I WILL DRINK ___ GLASSES OF WATER TODAY: 1 2 3 4 5 6 7 8 9 10

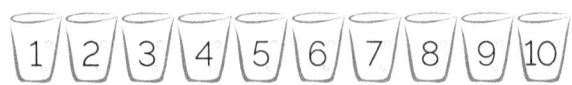

LOOKING BACK ON MY AMAZINGNESS

MY WINS I CELEBRATE TODAY ARE	TOMORROW I WILL IMPROVE ON

3 THINGS I AM THANKFUL FOR LAST 24 HOURS:

1. _____

2. _____

3. _____

THOUGHT DOWNLOAD

NOTES

AFFIRMATION OF THE DAY: _____

TODAY, I AM LOOKING FORWARD TO

GOALS #1	GOALS #2

HABITS I AM TRACKING	Y/N

THOUGHT DOWNLOAD

TODAY I AM CHOOSING TO FEEL:

C -

T -

F -
A -

R -

I WILL DRINK ___ GLASSES OF WATER TODAY: 1 2 3 4 5 6 7 8 9 10

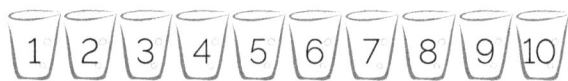

LOOKING BACK ON MY AMAZINGNESS

MY WINS I CELEBRATE TODAY ARE	TOMORROW I WILL IMPROVE ON

3 THINGS I AM THANKFUL FOR LAST 24 HOURS:

1. ______________________________

2. ______________________________

3. ______________________________

THOUGHT DOWNLOAD

NOTES

AFFIRMATION OF THE DAY: _____

TODAY, I AM LOOKING FORWARD TO

GOALS #1	GOALS #2	HABITS I AM TRACKING	Y/N

THOUGHT DOWNLOAD

TODAY I AM CHOOSING TO FEEL:

C -

T -

F -
A -

R -

I WILL DRINK ___ GLASSES OF WATER TODAY: 1 2 3 4 5 6 7 8 9 10

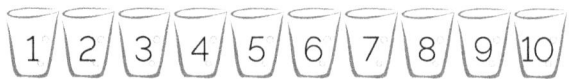

LOOKING BACK ON MY AMAZINGNESS

MY WINS I CELEBRATE TODAY ARE	TOMORROW I WILL IMPROVE ON

3 THINGS I AM THANKFUL FOR LAST 24 HOURS:

1. ______________________________

2. ______________________________

3. ______________________________

THOUGHT DOWNLOAD

NOTES

AFFIRMATION OF THE DAY: _____

TODAY, I AM LOOKING FORWARD TO

GOALS #1	GOALS #2	HABITS I AM TRACKING	Y/N

THOUGHT DOWNLOAD

TODAY I AM CHOOSING TO FEEL:

C -

T -

F -
A -

R -

I WILL DRINK ____ GLASSES OF WATER TODAY: 1 2 3 4 5 6 7 8 9 10

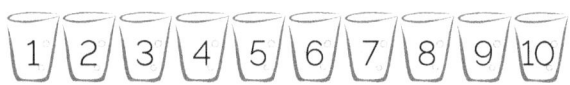

LOOKING BACK ON MY AMAZINGNESS

MY WINS I CELEBRATE TODAY ARE	TOMORROW I WILL IMPROVE ON

3 THINGS I AM THANKFUL FOR LAST 24 HOURS:

1. ______________________________

2. ______________________________

3. ______________________________

THOUGHT DOWNLOAD

NOTES

AFFIRMATION OF THE DAY: _____

TODAY, I AM LOOKING FORWARD TO

GOALS #1	GOALS #2	HABITS I AM TRACKING	Y/N

THOUGHT DOWNLOAD

TODAY I AM CHOOSING TO FEEL:

C -

T -

F -
A -

R -

I WILL DRINK ____ GLASSES OF WATER TODAY: 1 2 3 4 5 6 7 8 9 10

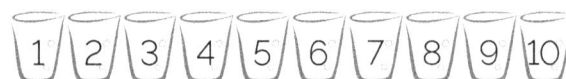

LOOKING BACK ON MY AMAZINGNESS

MY WINS I CELEBRATE TODAY ARE	TOMORROW I WILL IMPROVE ON

3 THINGS I AM THANKFUL FOR LAST 24 HOURS:

1. ____________________

2. ____________________

3. ____________________

THOUGHT DOWNLOAD

NOTES

AFFIRMATION OF THE DAY: _____

TODAY, I AM LOOKING FORWARD TO

GOALS #1	GOALS #2	HABITS I AM TRACKING	Y/N

THOUGHT DOWNLOAD

TODAY I AM CHOOSING TO FEEL:

C -

T -

F -
A -

R -

I WILL DRINK ___ GLASSES OF WATER TODAY: 1 2 3 4 5 6 7 8 9 10

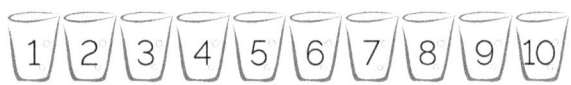

LOOKING BACK ON MY AMAZINGNESS

MY WINS I CELEBRATE TODAY ARE	TOMORROW I WILL IMPROVE ON

3 THINGS I AM THANKFUL FOR LAST 24 HOURS:

1. ______________________________

2. ______________________________

3. ______________________________

THOUGHT DOWNLOAD

NOTES

AFFIRMATION OF THE DAY: _____

TODAY, I AM LOOKING FORWARD TO

GOALS #1	GOALS #2	HABITS I AM TRACKING	Y/N

THOUGHT DOWNLOAD

TODAY I AM CHOOSING TO FEEL:

C -

T -

F -
A -

R -

I WILL DRINK ____ GLASSES OF WATER TODAY: 1 2 3 4 5 6 7 8 9 10

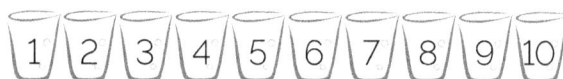

LOOKING BACK ON MY AMAZINGNESS

MY WINS I CELEBRATE TODAY ARE	TOMORROW I WILL IMPROVE ON

3 THINGS I AM THANKFUL FOR LAST 24 HOURS:

1. ______________________________

2. ______________________________

3. ______________________________

THOUGHT DOWNLOAD

NOTES

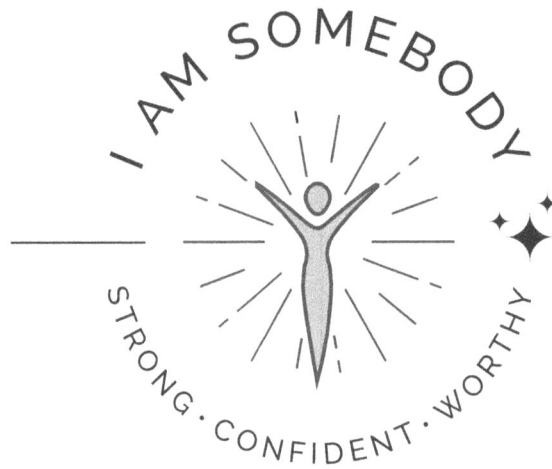

I AM SOMBODY

Transform Your Life Organizer™

Month Two

LIMITING BELIEFS

(Thoughts that limit you in some way from fulfilling your true potential or having all that you want in life).

DISPUTE NEGATIVE THINKING. We are going to first identify our thoughts and then decide if they are true. Is there evidence to support our beliefs?

If our beliefs are not true, we must replace them with new ones and one way to do that is to use affirmations and by repeating our new beliefs. Each day, there is a space in your organizer to write down an affirmation, but I also want you to look in the mirror and tell yourself that affirmation, for example, if you write **I AM Somebody**, look in the mirror and with belief and great feeling say **I Am Somebody**! You may want to repeat this as the day goes on, every time you see a mirror, remind yourself **I Am Somebody.**

People who have positive self-esteem tend to have an easier time dealing with whatever life throws at them. When we feel we have value and worth, we are better able to cope with life's challenges and traumas and we have a better chance of staying focused and moving forward.

It can be uncomfortable at first going through the process, hell, who am I kidding? The entire process has its uncomfortable moments but believe me, it is well worth it. YOU ARE WORTH IT! YOU ARE SOMEBODY!

Focus and believe that you are worthy, and I promise you can expect to receive improvements in all aspects of your life.

We are born knowing our self-worth, however as we get older, our sense of self-worth may not be intact due to other people's comments, expectations, and attitudes towards us. We can restore our sense of worth, but we cannot do it by turning to other people or external factors. If you ever built your happiness on another human's approval, behavior, the permanence of a relationship, or on certain material possessions, then you know it does not work. If I am basing my self worth on how much I can lift and then someone comes along my size and can lift heavier, then what happens? I begin to think I am not as strong as I thought, I should be lifting heavier, that person is better than me, etc. and my self worth begins to decrease. If I were basing my happiness on the approval of a loan to become a certified life coach through The Life Coach School then when I got denied, I would have been devastated, depressed and my whole feel-good attitude would have vanished. If the external factor changes then so does your happiness. We do not want to have our life fall apart or we do not want to question our worth, question our capabilities or what we deserve based on whether someone leaves us or whether we receive a promotion. This is when our self confidence begins to decrease and we stop acting, stop speaking up and taking chances. We can not let our happiness be the result of an outside factor.

SAY GOODBYE TO THOSE LIMITING BELIEFS THAT HAVE BEEN HOLDING YOU BACK!

BE UNSTOPPABLE

Ready to get rid of all those limiting beliefs that have been keeping you from living your happiest life? You can use this worksheet to get rid of any limiting thoughts about any topic you like. Since we are working on our Self Worth, we are going to choose that limiting belief today.

Step 1: The topic we want to clear our limiting beliefs around is **SELF WORTH**

Step 2: In column one, write down a list of limiting beliefs you have around this topic, such as I am not loveable, I cannot do anything right, it is all my parents' fault, I am not worth it, I am a waste of space, I am a failure, etc....

TOPIC: SELF WORTH

STEP 2	STEP 3	STEP 6
LIST OF LIMITING BELIEFS	**ARE THESE BELIEFS TRUE- WHY/WHY NOT?**	**NEW BELIEFS AND THE FACTS TO PROVE**
I am not worthy of good things.	No, because we are all born worthy.	Things do not define my worth.

Step 3: Read your limiting beliefs from column one out loud, are any of these beliefs true? Which, if any, are facts, not thoughts or judgements? In column two, write whether the limiting beliefs are true or not and why. Now repeat them out loud.

Step 4: Forgive yourself or others for all the different limiting beliefs you have developed.

Step 5: Imagine being free and give yourself permission to honor your limiting beliefs and move past them. Say this out loud… **"I give myself permission to let go of believing that I am not worthy, and I am ready to replace it with I am worthy. This has been holding me back and I am looking forward to seeing and feeling all the new possibilities and opportunities ahead of me."**

Step 6: In column 3, write down your new beliefs compared to your column 2, I no longer believe I am not loveable; I am choosing to replace it with I am loveable. Then write the evidence to back it up. Keep adding to this list, why you are loved until you genuinely believe it.

EVEN IF YOU DO NOT BELIEVE YOU ARE WORTH IT,

GUESS WHAT... YOU STILL ARE WORTHY!

We are usually our biggest critic especially when faced with a difficult situation or when speaking of ourselves. Words are as powerful as they can uplift or destroy, they can trigger memories of success or failure and depending on how we think, it can significantly affect how we handle challenges.

TASK: Complete the following exercise once daily for the first Week of this month.

Pay attention and as you notice yourself participating in the negative self talk, I want you to acknowledge that it is what you are doing and then replace it with the positive equivalent. Remember, you must not judge negative self-talk and you must believe in the positive equivalent. On the left-hand side write out your negative thoughts that you have about yourself or your life, an example is given.

Identify and then challenge your negative beliefs about yourself. Notice your thoughts about yourself. You might find yourself thinking, 'I'm not clever enough to do that' or 'I have no friends.' When you do, look for evidence that contradicts those statements. Write down both statement and evidence and keep looking back at it to remind yourself that your negative beliefs about yourself are not true. No matter what, do not judge yourself or your thoughts.

TYPICAL NEGATIVE THOUGHTS	DISPUTE NEGATIVE THOUGHT
I cannot do this; I am going to fail.	I will put in an effort, that alone is a pass in my books.

TASK: Complete the following exercise once for the next 7 days or you can put one in each day for the next 7 days.

Pay attention to the negative thoughts that you have about others or life in general, an example is done for you.

Assess each thought individually, read each out loud and then I want you to dispute it in the column beside it with a statement that you believe. No matter what, do not judge yourself or your thoughts.

TYPICAL NEGATIVE THOUGHTS	DISPUTE NEGATIVE THOUGHT
I cannot do this; I am going to fail.	I will put in an effort, that alone is a pass in my books.

MONTHLY GOALS

WOO-HOO LOOK AT YOU GO:

"It is never too late to be what you might have been" George Eliot

6 MONTHS GOAL	MONTHLY GOAL
GOAL #1	
GOAL #2	

MONTH AT A GLANCE -

TAKE THIS MONTH BY THE HORNS AND GIVE IT YOUR ALL

NOTES			

YOU ARE STRONGER THAN YOUR BIGGEST STRUGGLE!

Every Sunday review & re-evaluate your goals. Identify obstacles that you faced, along with solutions.

	START CHANGING THE STORY YOU TELL YOURSELF.	INSTEAD OF AUTOMATICALLY THINKING YOU CAN'T DO SOMETHING, SAY "I HAVE NEVER DONE IT, BUT I WILL GIVE IT A TRY."	Say it with me... I AM SOMEBODY

MY WEEK OF AWESOMENESS!
Now that 6 month and monthly goals are done, we now can break down
our goals even further to make them even more achievable

REFLECTIONS OF LAST WEEK:

OBSTACLES I MAY FACE: _____

_____

SOLUTIONS: _____

_____

MY WEEK OF_____
Take 1-5 days this month to go through all your belongings and what you do not use regularly or have multiple of them is time to part with them. When parting with anything that is not actual trash, donate or sell these items.

TIME			

JENNIFER BULBROOK

MY WEEK OF AWESOMENESS!

6 Month Goal	6 Month Goal
MONTH	MONTH
WEEK	WEEK
REWARD WHEN I REACH	REWARD WHEN I REACH

MY WEEK OF_____
What time do you want to wake up at, go to bed? How do you want your week to look like?
What events or meetings do you need to attend? Are you planning on having a day of shopping?

AFFIRMATION OF THE DAY: _____

TODAY, I AM LOOKING FORWARD TO

GOALS #1	GOALS #2	HABITS I AM TRACKING	Y/N

THOUGHT DOWNLOAD

TODAY I AM CHOOSING TO FEEL:

C -

T -

F -
A -

R -

I WILL DRINK ____ GLASSES OF WATER TODAY: 1 2 3 4 5 6 7 8 9 10

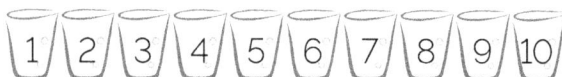

LOOKING BACK ON MY AMAZINGNESS

MY WINS I CELEBRATE TODAY ARE	TOMORROW I WILL IMPROVE ON

3 THINGS I AM THANKFUL FOR LAST 24 HOURS:

1. ____________________

2. ____________________

3. ____________________

THOUGHT DOWNLOAD

NOTES

AFFIRMATION OF THE DAY: _____

TODAY, I AM LOOKING FORWARD TO

GOALS #1	GOALS #2	HABITS I AM TRACKING	Y/N

THOUGHT DOWNLOAD

TODAY I AM CHOOSING TO FEEL:

C -

T -

F -
A -

R -

I WILL DRINK ___ GLASSES OF WATER TODAY: 1 2 3 4 5 6 7 8 9 10

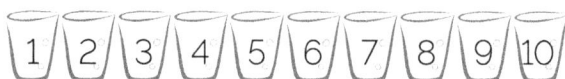

LOOKING BACK ON MY AMAZINGNESS

MY WINS I CELEBRATE TODAY ARE	TOMORROW I WILL IMPROVE ON

3 THINGS I AM THANKFUL FOR LAST 24 HOURS:

1. ______________________________

2. ______________________________

3. ______________________________

THOUGHT DOWNLOAD

NOTES

AFFIRMATION OF THE DAY: _

TODAY, I AM LOOKING FORWARD TO

GOALS #1	GOALS #2	HABITS I AM TRACKING	Y/N

THOUGHT DOWNLOAD

TODAY I AM CHOOSING TO FEEL:

C -

T -

F -
A -

R -

I WILL DRINK ____ GLASSES OF WATER TODAY: 1 2 3 4 5 6 7 8 9 10

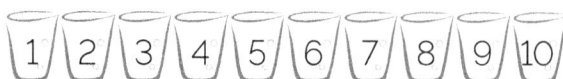

LOOKING BACK ON MY AMAZINGNESS

MY WINS I CELEBRATE TODAY ARE	TOMORROW I WILL IMPROVE ON

3 THINGS I AM THANKFUL FOR LAST 24 HOURS:

1. ______________________________

2. ______________________________

3. ______________________________

THOUGHT DOWNLOAD

NOTES

AFFIRMATION OF THE DAY: _____

TODAY, I AM LOOKING FORWARD TO

GOALS #1	GOALS #2	HABITS I AM TRACKING	Y/N

THOUGHT DOWNLOAD

TODAY I AM CHOOSING TO FEEL:

C -

T -

F -
A -

R -

I WILL DRINK ___ GLASSES OF WATER TODAY: 1 2 3 4 5 6 7 8 9 10

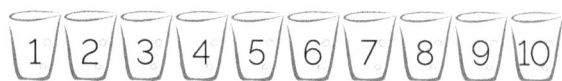

LOOKING BACK ON MY AMAZINGNESS

MY WINS I CELEBRATE TODAY ARE	TOMORROW I WILL IMPROVE ON

3 THINGS I AM THANKFUL FOR LAST 24 HOURS:

1. ______________________________

2. ______________________________

3. ______________________________

THOUGHT DOWNLOAD

NOTES

AFFIRMATION OF THE DAY: _____

TODAY, I AM LOOKING FORWARD TO

GOALS #1	GOALS #2	HABITS I AM TRACKING	Y/N

THOUGHT DOWNLOAD

TODAY I AM CHOOSING TO FEEL:

C -

T -

F -
A -

R -

I WILL DRINK ___ GLASSES OF WATER TODAY: 1 2 3 4 5 6 7 8 9 10

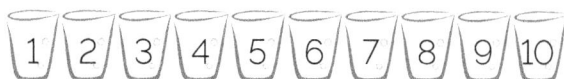

LOOKING BACK ON MY AMAZINGNESS

MY WINS I CELEBRATE TODAY ARE	TOMORROW I WILL IMPROVE ON

3 THINGS I AM THANKFUL FOR LAST 24 HOURS:

1. ______________________________

2. ______________________________

3. ______________________________

THOUGHT DOWNLOAD

NOTES

AFFIRMATION OF THE DAY: _____

TODAY, I AM LOOKING FORWARD TO

GOALS #1	GOALS #2	HABITS I AM TRACKING	Y/N

THOUGHT DOWNLOAD

TODAY I AM CHOOSING TO FEEL:

C -

T -

F -
A -

R -

I WILL DRINK ___ GLASSES OF WATER TODAY: 1 2 3 4 5 6 7 8 9 10

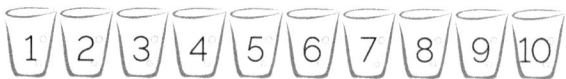

LOOKING BACK ON MY AMAZINGNESS

MY WINS I CELEBRATE TODAY ARE	TOMORROW I WILL IMPROVE ON

3 THINGS I AM THANKFUL FOR LAST 24 HOURS:

1. ______________________________

2. ______________________________

3. ______________________________

THOUGHT DOWNLOAD

NOTES

AFFIRMATION OF THE DAY: _

TODAY, I AM LOOKING FORWARD TO

GOALS #1	GOALS #2	HABITS I AM TRACKING	Y/N

THOUGHT DOWNLOAD

TODAY I AM CHOOSING TO FEEL:

C -

T -

F -
A -

R -

I WILL DRINK ___ GLASSES OF WATER TODAY: 1 2 3 4 5 6 7 8 9 10

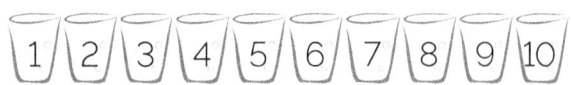

JENNIFER BULBROOK

LOOKING BACK ON MY AMAZINGNESS

MY WINS I CELEBRATE TODAY ARE	TOMORROW I WILL IMPROVE ON

3 THINGS I AM THANKFUL FOR LAST 24 HOURS:

1. _____

2. _____

3. _____

THOUGHT DOWNLOAD

NOTES

MY WEEK OF AWESOMENESS!
Now that 6 month and monthly goals are done, we now can break down
our goals even further to make them even more achievable

REFLECTIONS OF LAST WEEK:

OBSTACLES I MAY FACE: _____

_____

SOLUTIONS: _____

_____

MY WEEK OF_____
Take 1-5 days this month to go through all your belongings and what you do not use regularly or have multiple of them is time to part with them. When parting with anything that is not actual trash, donate or sell these items.

TIME			

JENNIFER BULBROOK

MY WEEK OF AWESOMENESS!

6 Month Goal	6 Month Goal
MONTH	MONTH
WEEK	WEEK
REWARD WHEN I REACH	REWARD WHEN I REACH

MY WEEK OF_____

What time do you want to wake up at, go to bed? How do you want your week to look like?

What events or meetings do you need to attend? Are you planning on having a day of shopping?

I ACCEPT MYSELF!

AFFIRMATION OF THE DAY: _____

TODAY, I AM LOOKING FORWARD TO

GOALS #1

GOALS #2

HABITS I AM TRACKING	Y/N

THOUGHT DOWNLOAD

TODAY I AM CHOOSING TO FEEL:

C -

T -

F -
A -

R -

I WILL DRINK ___ GLASSES OF WATER TODAY: 1 2 3 4 5 6 7 8 9 10

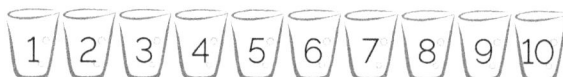

LOOKING BACK ON MY AMAZINGNESS

MY WINS I CELEBRATE TODAY ARE	TOMORROW I WILL IMPROVE ON

3 THINGS I AM THANKFUL FOR LAST 24 HOURS:

1. ______________________________

2. ______________________________

3. ______________________________

THOUGHT DOWNLOAD

NOTES

AFFIRMATION OF THE DAY: _____

TODAY, I AM LOOKING FORWARD TO

GOALS #1

GOALS #2

HABITS I AM TRACKING	Y/N

THOUGHT DOWNLOAD

TODAY I AM CHOOSING TO FEEL:

C -

T -

F -
A -

R -

I WILL DRINK ___ GLASSES OF WATER TODAY: 1 2 3 4 5 6 7 8 9 10

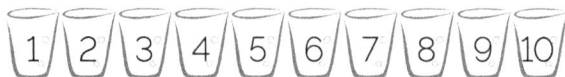

LOOKING BACK ON MY AMAZINGNESS

MY WINS I CELEBRATE TODAY ARE	TOMORROW I WILL IMPROVE ON

3 THINGS I AM THANKFUL FOR LAST 24 HOURS:

1. ____________________

2. ____________________

3. ____________________

THOUGHT DOWNLOAD

NOTES

AFFIRMATION OF THE DAY: _____

TODAY, I AM LOOKING FORWARD TO

GOALS #1	GOALS #2

HABITS I AM TRACKING	Y/N

THOUGHT DOWNLOAD

TODAY I AM CHOOSING TO FEEL:

C -

T -

F -
A -

R -

I WILL DRINK ___ GLASSES OF WATER TODAY: 1 2 3 4 5 6 7 8 9 10

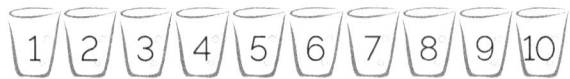

LOOKING BACK ON MY AMAZINGNESS

MY WINS I CELEBRATE TODAY ARE	TOMORROW I WILL IMPROVE ON

3 THINGS I AM THANKFUL FOR LAST 24 HOURS:

1. ______________________________

2. ______________________________

3. ______________________________

THOUGHT DOWNLOAD

NOTES

AFFIRMATION OF THE DAY: _____

TODAY, I AM LOOKING FORWARD TO

GOALS #1	GOALS #2	HABITS I AM TRACKING	Y/N

THOUGHT DOWNLOAD

TODAY I AM CHOOSING TO FEEL:

C -

T -

F -

A -

R -

I WILL DRINK ____ GLASSES OF WATER TODAY: 1 2 3 4 5 6 7 8 9 10

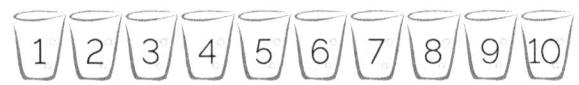

LOOKING BACK ON MY AMAZINGNESS

MY WINS I CELEBRATE TODAY ARE	TOMORROW I WILL IMPROVE ON

3 THINGS I AM THANKFUL FOR LAST 24 HOURS:

1. ______________________________

2. ______________________________

3. ______________________________

THOUGHT DOWNLOAD

NOTES

AFFIRMATION OF THE DAY: _____

TODAY, I AM LOOKING FORWARD TO

GOALS #1	GOALS #2	HABITS I AM TRACKING	Y/N

THOUGHT DOWNLOAD

TODAY I AM CHOOSING TO FEEL:

C -

T -

F -
A -

R -

I WILL DRINK ___ GLASSES OF WATER TODAY: 1 2 3 4 5 6 7 8 9 10

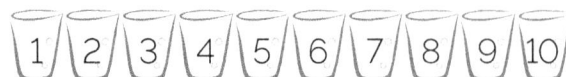

LOOKING BACK ON MY AMAZINGNESS

MY WINS I CELEBRATE TODAY ARE	TOMORROW I WILL IMPROVE ON

3 THINGS I AM THANKFUL FOR LAST 24 HOURS:

1. _____

2. _____

3. _____

THOUGHT DOWNLOAD

NOTES

AFFIRMATION OF THE DAY: _____

TODAY, I AM LOOKING FORWARD TO

GOALS #1	GOALS #2	HABITS I AM TRACKING	Y/N

THOUGHT DOWNLOAD

TODAY I AM CHOOSING TO FEEL:

C -

T -

F -
A -

R -

I WILL DRINK ___ GLASSES OF WATER TODAY: 1 2 3 4 5 6 7 8 9 10

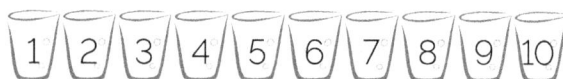

LOOKING BACK ON MY AMAZINGNESS

MY WINS I CELEBRATE TODAY ARE	TOMORROW I WILL IMPROVE ON

3 THINGS I AM THANKFUL FOR LAST 24 HOURS:

1. ______________________________

2. ______________________________

3. ______________________________

THOUGHT DOWNLOAD

NOTES

AFFIRMATION OF THE DAY: _

TODAY, I AM LOOKING FORWARD TO

GOALS #1	GOALS #2	HABITS I AM TRACKING	Y/N

THOUGHT DOWNLOAD

TODAY I AM CHOOSING TO FEEL:

C -

T -

F -
A -

R -

I WILL DRINK ___ GLASSES OF WATER TODAY: 1 2 3 4 5 6 7 8 9 10

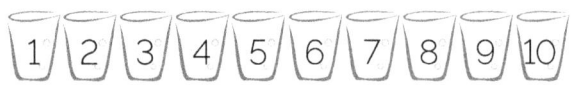

LOOKING BACK ON MY AMAZINGNESS

MY WINS I CELEBRATE TODAY ARE	TOMORROW I WILL IMPROVE ON

3 THINGS I AM THANKFUL FOR LAST 24 HOURS:

1. _____

2. _____

3. _____

THOUGHT DOWNLOAD

NOTES

MY WEEK OF AWESOMENESS!
Now that 6 month and monthly goals are done, we now can break down
our goals even further to make them even more achievable

REFLECTIONS OF LAST WEEK:

OBSTACLES I MAY FACE: _____

_____

SOLUTIONS: _____

_____

MY WEEK OF_____
Take 1-5 days this month to go through all your belongings and what you do not use regularly or have multiple of them is time to part with them. When parting with anything that is not actual trash, donate or sell these items.

TIME			

MY WEEK OF AWESOMENESS!

6 Month Goal	6 Month Goal
MONTH	MONTH
WEEK	WEEK
REWARD WHEN I REACH	REWARD WHEN I REACH

MY WEEK OF_____

What time do you want to wake up at, go to bed? How do you want your week to look like?

What events or meetings do you need to attend? Are you planning on having a day of shopping?

AFFIRMATION OF THE DAY: _____

TODAY, I AM LOOKING FORWARD TO

GOALS #1	GOALS #2	HABITS I AM TRACKING	Y/N

THOUGHT DOWNLOAD

TODAY I AM CHOOSING TO FEEL:

C -

T -

F -
A -

R -

I WILL DRINK ___ GLASSES OF WATER TODAY: 1 2 3 4 5 6 7 8 9 10

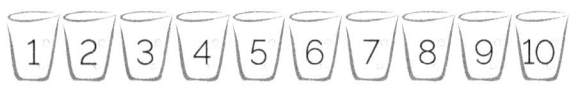

LOOKING BACK ON MY AMAZINGNESS

MY WINS I CELEBRATE TODAY ARE	TOMORROW I WILL IMPROVE ON

3 THINGS I AM THANKFUL FOR LAST 24 HOURS:

1. ______________________________

2. ______________________________

3. ______________________________

THOUGHT DOWNLOAD

NOTES

AFFIRMATION OF THE DAY: --

TODAY, I AM LOOKING FORWARD TO

GOALS #1	GOALS #2	HABITS I AM TRACKING	Y/N

THOUGHT DOWNLOAD

TODAY I AM CHOOSING TO FEEL:

C -

T -

F -
A -

R -

I WILL DRINK ___ GLASSES OF WATER TODAY: 1 2 3 4 5 6 7 8 9 10

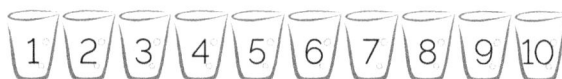

LOOKING BACK ON MY AMAZINGNESS

MY WINS I CELEBRATE TODAY ARE	TOMORROW I WILL IMPROVE ON

3 THINGS I AM THANKFUL FOR LAST 24 HOURS:

1. ______________________________

2. ______________________________

3. ______________________________

THOUGHT DOWNLOAD

NOTES

AFFIRMATION OF THE DAY: _

TODAY, I AM LOOKING FORWARD TO

GOALS #1	GOALS #2

HABITS I AM TRACKING	Y/N

THOUGHT DOWNLOAD

TODAY I AM CHOOSING TO FEEL:

C -

T -

F -
A -

R -

I WILL DRINK ___ GLASSES OF WATER TODAY: 1 2 3 4 5 6 7 8 9 10

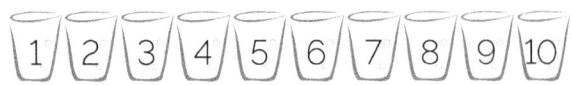

LOOKING BACK ON MY AMAZINGNESS

MY WINS I CELEBRATE TODAY ARE	TOMORROW I WILL IMPROVE ON

3 THINGS I AM THANKFUL FOR LAST 24 HOURS:

1. ______________________________

2. ______________________________

3. ______________________________

THOUGHT DOWNLOAD

NOTES

I AM GRATEFUL!

AFFIRMATION OF THE DAY: _____

TODpAY, I AM LOOKING FORWARD TO

GOALS #1	GOALS #2	HABITS I AM TRACKING	Y/N

THOUGHT DOWNLOAD

TODAY I AM CHOOSING TO FEEL:

C -

T -

F -
A -

R -

I WILL DRINK ___ GLASSES OF WATER TODAY: 1 2 3 4 5 6 7 8 9 10

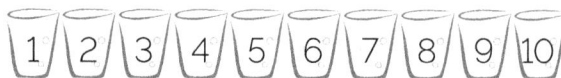

LOOKING BACK ON MY AMAZINGNESS

MY WINS I CELEBRATE TODAY ARE	TOMORROW I WILL IMPROVE ON

3 THINGS I AM THANKFUL FOR LAST 24 HOURS:

1. ______________________________

2. ______________________________

3. ______________________________

THOUGHT DOWNLOAD

NOTES

AFFIRMATION OF THE DAY: _____

TODAY, I AM LOOKING FORWARD TO

GOALS #1	GOALS #2	HABITS I AM TRACKING	Y/N

THOUGHT DOWNLOAD

TODAY I AM CHOOSING TO FEEL:

C -

T -

F -
A -

R -

I WILL DRINK ___ GLASSES OF WATER TODAY: 1 2 3 4 5 6 7 8 9 10

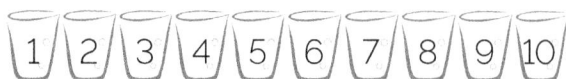

LOOKING BACK ON MY AMAZINGNESS

MY WINS I CELEBRATE TODAY ARE	TOMORROW I WILL IMPROVE ON

3 THINGS I AM THANKFUL FOR LAST 24 HOURS:

1. ________________

2. ________________

3. ________________

THOUGHT DOWNLOAD

NOTES

AFFIRMATION OF THE DAY: _____

TODAY, I AM LOOKING FORWARD TO

GOALS #1	GOALS #2	HABITS I AM TRACKING	Y/N

THOUGHT DOWNLOAD

TODAY I AM CHOOSING TO FEEL:

C -

T -

F -
A -

R -

I WILL DRINK ____ GLASSES OF WATER TODAY: 1 2 3 4 5 6 7 8 9 10

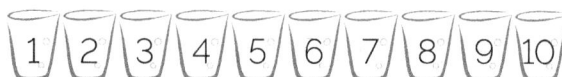

LOOKING BACK ON MY AMAZINGNESS

MY WINS I CELEBRATE TODAY ARE	TOMORROW I WILL IMPROVE ON

3 THINGS I AM THANKFUL FOR LAST 24 HOURS:

1. ______________________________

2. ______________________________

3. ______________________________

THOUGHT DOWNLOAD

NOTES

AFFIRMATION OF THE DAY: _____

TODAY, I AM LOOKING FORWARD TO

GOALS #1	GOALS #2	HABITS I AM TRACKING	Y/N

THOUGHT DOWNLOAD

TODAY I AM CHOOSING TO FEEL:

C -

T -

F -
A -

R -

I WILL DRINK ___ GLASSES OF WATER TODAY: 1 2 3 4 5 6 7 8 9 10

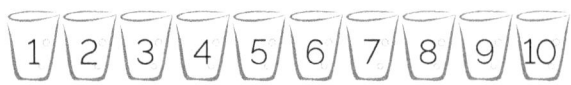

LOOKING BACK ON MY AMAZINGNESS

MY WINS I CELEBRATE TODAY ARE	TOMORROW I WILL IMPROVE ON

3 THINGS I AM THANKFUL FOR LAST 24 HOURS:

1. --

2. --

3. --

THOUGHT DOWNLOAD

NOTES

MY WEEK OF AWESOMENESS!
**Now that 6 month and monthly goals are done, we now can break down
our goals even further to make them even more achievable**

REFLECTIONS OF LAST WEEK:

OBSTACLES I MAY FACE: _____

_____

SOLUTIONS: _____

_____

MY WEEK OF_____
**Take 1-5 days this month to go through all your belongings and what you do not use regularly or have multiple of
them is time to part with them. When parting with anything that is not actual trash, donate or sell these items.**

TIME			

JENNIFER BULBROOK

MY WEEK OF AWESOMENESS!

6 Month Goal	6 Month Goal
MONTH	MONTH
WEEK	WEEK
REWARD WHEN REACH	REWARD WHEN REACH

MY WEEK OF_____

What time do you want to wake up at, go to bed? How do you want your week to look like?

What events or meetings do you need to attend? Are you planning on having a day of shopping?

AFFIRMATION OF THE DAY: _____

TODAY, I AM LOOKING FORWARD TO

GOALS #1	GOALS #2	HABITS I AM TRACKING	Y/N

THOUGHT DOWNLOAD

TODAY I AM CHOOSING TO FEEL:

C -

T -

F -
A -

R -

I WILL DRINK ___ GLASSES OF WATER TODAY: 1 2 3 4 5 6 7 8 9 10

LOOKING BACK ON MY AMAZINGNESS

MY WINS I CELEBRATE TODAY ARE	TOMORROW I WILL IMPROVE ON

3 THINGS I AM THANKFUL FOR LAST 24 HOURS:

1. ______________________________

2. ______________________________

3. ______________________________

THOUGHT DOWNLOAD

NOTES

AFFIRMATION OF THE DAY: _____

TODAY, I AM LOOKING FORWARD TO

GOALS #1	GOALS #2	HABITS I AM TRACKING	Y/N

THOUGHT DOWNLOAD

TODAY I AM CHOOSING TO FEEL:

C -

T -

F -
A -

R -

I WILL DRINK ___ GLASSES OF WATER TODAY: 1 2 3 4 5 6 7 8 9 10

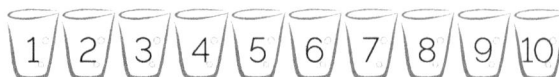

LOOKING BACK ON MY AMAZINGNESS

MY WINS I CELEBRATE TODAY ARE	TOMORROW I WILL IMPROVE ON

3 THINGS I AM THANKFUL FOR LAST 24 HOURS:

1. ______________________________

2. ______________________________

3. ______________________________

THOUGHT DOWNLOAD

NOTES

AFFIRMATION OF THE DAY: _____

TODAY, I AM LOOKING FORWARD TO

GOALS #1	GOALS #2	HABITS I AM TRACKING	Y/N

THOUGHT DOWNLOAD

TODAY I AM CHOOSING TO FEEL:

C -

T -

F -
A -

R -

I WILL DRINK ___ GLASSES OF WATER TODAY: 1 2 3 4 5 6 7 8 9 10

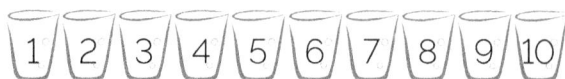

LOOKING BACK ON MY AMAZINGNESS

MY WINS I CELEBRATE TODAY ARE	TOMORROW I WILL IMPROVE ON

3 THINGS I AM THANKFUL FOR LAST 24 HOURS:

1. ______________________________

2. ______________________________

3. ______________________________

THOUGHT DOWNLOAD

NOTES

AFFIRMATION OF THE DAY: _____

TODAY, I AM LOOKING FORWARD TO

GOALS #1	GOALS #2	HABITS I AM TRACKING	Y/N

THOUGHT DOWNLOAD

TODAY I AM CHOOSING TO FEEL:

C -

T -

F -
A -

R -

I WILL DRINK ___ GLASSES OF WATER TODAY: 1 2 3 4 5 6 7 8 9 10

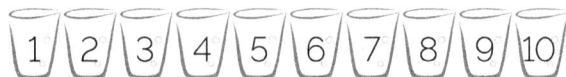

LOOKING BACK ON MY AMAZINGNESS

MY WINS I CELEBRATE TODAY ARE	TOMORROW I WILL IMPROVE ON

3 THINGS I AM THANKFUL FOR LAST 24 HOURS:

1. ______________________________

2. ______________________________

3. ______________________________

THOUGHT DOWNLOAD

NOTES

AFFIRMATION OF THE DAY: _____

TODAY, I AM LOOKING FORWARD TO

GOALS #1	GOALS #2	HABITS I AM TRACKING	Y/N

THOUGHT DOWNLOAD

TODAY I AM CHOOSING TO FEEL:

C -

T -

F -
A -

R -

I WILL DRINK ___ GLASSES OF WATER TODAY: 1 2 3 4 5 6 7 8 9 10

LOOKING BACK ON MY AMAZINGNESS

MY WINS I CELEBRATE TODAY ARE	TOMORROW I WILL IMPROVE ON

3 THINGS I AM THANKFUL FOR LAST 24 HOURS:

1. ______________________________

2. ______________________________

3. ______________________________

THOUGHT DOWNLOAD

NOTES

I AM WORTHY!

AFFIRMATION OF THE DAY: _____

TODAY, I AM LOOKING FORWARD TO

GOALS #1   GOALS #2   HABITS I AM TRACKING   Y/N

THOUGHT DOWNLOAD

TODAY I AM CHOOSING TO FEEL:

C -

T -

F -
A -

R -

I WILL DRINK ___ GLASSES OF WATER TODAY: 1 2 3 4 5 6 7 8 9 10

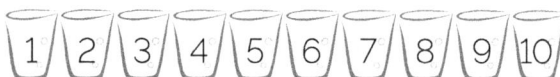

LOOKING BACK ON MY AMAZINGNESS

MY WINS I CELEBRATE TODAY ARE	TOMORROW I WILL IMPROVE ON

3 THINGS I AM THANKFUL FOR LAST 24 HOURS:

1. ______________________________

2. ______________________________

3. ______________________________

THOUGHT DOWNLOAD

NOTES

AFFIRMATION OF THE DAY: --

TODAY, I AM LOOKING FORWARD TO

GOALS #1	GOALS #2	HABITS I AM TRACKING	Y/N

THOUGHT DOWNLOAD

TODAY I AM CHOOSING TO FEEL:

C -

T -

F -
A -

R -

I WILL DRINK ___ GLASSES OF WATER TODAY: 1 2 3 4 5 6 7 8 9 10

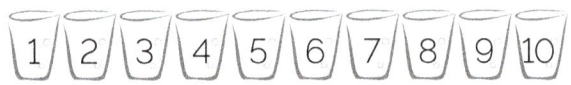

LOOKING BACK ON MY AMAZINGNESS

MY WINS I CELEBRATE TODAY ARE	TOMORROW I WILL IMPROVE ON

3 THINGS I AM THANKFUL FOR LAST 24 HOURS:

1. _____

2. _____

3. _____

THOUGHT DOWNLOAD

NOTES

MY WEEK OF AWESOMENESS!
Now that 6 month and monthly goals are done, we now can break down
our goals even further to make them even more achievable

REFLECTIONS OF LAST WEEK:

OBSTACLES I MAY FACE: _____

_____

SOLUTIONS: _____

_____

MY WEEK OF_____
Take 1-5 days this month to go through all your belongings and what you do not use regularly or have multiple of
them is time to part with them. When parting with anything that is not actual trash, donate or sell these items.

TIME			

MY WEEK OF AWESOMENESS!

6 Month Goal	6 Month Goal
MONTH	MONTH
WEEK	WEEK
REWARD WHEN I REACH	REWARD WHEN I REACH

MY WEEK OF_____

What time do you want to wake up at, go to bed? How do you want your week to look like?

What events or meetings do you need to attend? Are you planning on having a day of shopping?

AFFIRMATION OF THE DAY: _____

TODAY, I AM LOOKING FORWARD TO

GOALS #1	GOALS #2	HABITS I AM TRACKING	Y/N

THOUGHT DOWNLOAD

TODAY I AM CHOOSING TO FEEL:

C -

T -

F -
A -

R -

I WILL DRINK ___ GLASSES OF WATER TODAY: 1 2 3 4 5 6 7 8 9 10

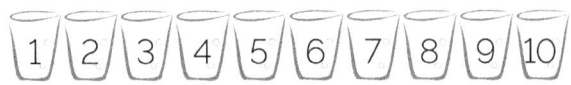

LOOKING BACK ON MY AMAZINGNESS

MY WINS I CELEBRATE TODAY ARE	TOMORROW I WILL IMPROVE ON

3 THINGS I AM THANKFUL FOR LAST 24 HOURS:

1. ____________________
2. ____________________
3. ____________________

THOUGHT DOWNLOAD

NOTES

AFFIRMATION OF THE DAY: _____

TODAY, I AM LOOKING FORWARD TO

GOALS #1	GOALS #2

HABITS I AM TRACKING	Y/N

THOUGHT DOWNLOAD

TODAY I AM CHOOSING TO FEEL:

C -

T -

F -
A -

R -

I WILL DRINK ____ GLASSES OF WATER TODAY: 1 2 3 4 5 6 7 8 9 10

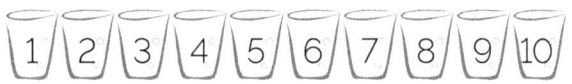

LOOKING BACK ON MY AMAZINGNESS

MY WINS I CELEBRATE TODAY ARE	TOMORROW I WILL IMPROVE ON

3 THINGS I AM THANKFUL FOR LAST 24 HOURS:

1. ______

2. ______

3. ______

THOUGHT DOWNLOAD

NOTES

AFFIRMATION OF THE DAY: _

TODAY, I AM LOOKING FORWARD TO

GOALS #1	GOALS #2	HABITS I AM TRACKING	Y/N

THOUGHT DOWNLOAD

TODAY I AM CHOOSING TO FEEL:

C -

T -

F -
A -

R -

I WILL DRINK ___ GLASSES OF WATER TODAY: 1 2 3 4 5 6 7 8 9 10

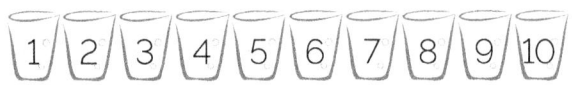

LOOKING BACK ON MY AMAZINGNESS

MY WINS I CELEBRATE TODAY ARE	TOMORROW I WILL IMPROVE ON

3 THINGS I AM THANKFUL FOR LAST 24 HOURS:

1. _____

2. _____

3. _____

THOUGHT DOWNLOAD

NOTES

AFFIRMATION OF THE DAY: _____

TODAY, I AM LOOKING FORWARD TO

GOALS #1	GOALS #2	HABITS I AM TRACKING	Y/N

THOUGHT DOWNLOAD

TODAY I AM CHOOSING TO FEEL:

C -

T -

F -
A -

R -

I WILL DRINK ___ GLASSES OF WATER TODAY: 1 2 3 4 5 6 7 8 9 10

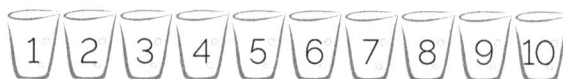

LOOKING BACK ON MY AMAZINGNESS

MY WINS I CELEBRATE TODAY ARE	TOMORROW I WILL IMPROVE ON

3 THINGS I AM THANKFUL FOR LAST 24 HOURS:

1. ______________________________

2. ______________________________

3. ______________________________

THOUGHT DOWNLOAD

NOTES

AFFIRMATION OF THE DAY: _____

TODAY, I AM LOOKING FORWARD TO

GOALS #1	GOALS #2	HABITS I AM TRACKING	Y/N

THOUGHT DOWNLOAD

TODAY I AM CHOOSING TO FEEL:

C -

T -

F -
A -

R -

I WILL DRINK ___ GLASSES OF WATER TODAY: 1 2 3 4 5 6 7 8 9 10

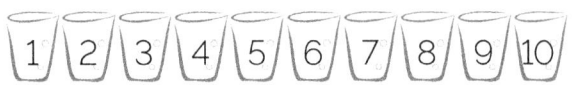

JENNIFER BULBROOK

LOOKING BACK ON MY AMAZINGNESS

MY WINS I CELEBRATE TODAY ARE	TOMORROW I WILL IMPROVE ON

3 THINGS I AM THANKFUL FOR LAST 24 HOURS:

1. ____________________

2. ____________________

3. ____________________

THOUGHT DOWNLOAD

NOTES

IF I AM SOMEBODY BELIEVES IN ME THEN I MUST BELIEVE IN ME!

AFFIRMATION OF THE DAY: _____

TODAY, I AM LOOKING FORWARD TO

GOALS #1	GOALS #2	HABITS I AM TRACKING	Y/N

THOUGHT DOWNLOAD

TODAY I AM CHOOSING TO FEEL:

C -

T -

F -
A -

R -

I WILL DRINK ___ GLASSES OF WATER TODAY: 1 2 3 4 5 6 7 8 9 10

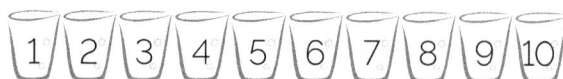

JENNIFER BULBROOK

LOOKING BACK ON MY AMAZINGNESS

MY WINS I CELEBRATE TODAY ARE	TOMORROW I WILL IMPROVE ON

3 THINGS I AM THANKFUL FOR LAST 24 HOURS:

1. ____

2. ____

3. ____

THOUGHT DOWNLOAD

NOTES

AFFIRMATION OF THE DAY: _____

TODAY, I AM LOOKING FORWARD TO

GOALS #1	GOALS #2	HABITS I AM TRACKING	Y/N

THOUGHT DOWNLOAD

TODAY I AM CHOOSING TO FEEL:

C -

T -

F -
A -

R -

I WILL DRINK ___ GLASSES OF WATER TODAY: 1 2 3 4 5 6 7 8 9 10

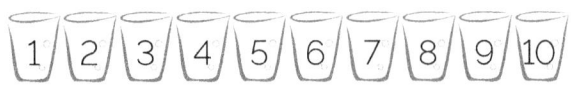

JENNIFER BULBROOK

LOOKING BACK ON MY AMAZINGNESS

MY WINS I CELEBRATE TODAY ARE	TOMORROW I WILL IMPROVE ON

3 THINGS I AM THANKFUL FOR LAST 24 HOURS:

1. ______________________________

2. ______________________________

3. ______________________________

THOUGHT DOWNLOAD

NOTES

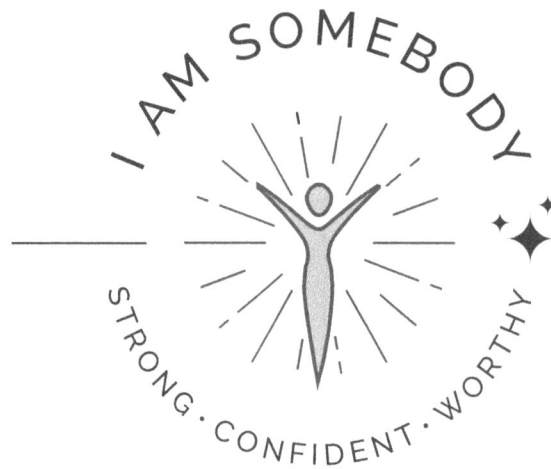

I AM SOMEBODY

STRONG · CONFIDENT · WORTHY

I AM SOMBODY

Transform Your Life Organizer™

Month Three

SELF-LOVE

Self-love is not about spa day, new outfits, or the sweet treats you have after dinner. These are just actual times when you show yourself some love.

"Self Love" refers to our ability to hold ourselves in esteem and have confidence in our worth, no matter what happens around us." www.growingself.com/what-is-self-love/

"Self-love means having a high regard for your own well-being and happiness. Self-love means taking care of your own needs and not sacrificing your well-being to please others. Self-love means not settling for less than you deserve." abrandtherapy.com/what-do-we-mean-when-we-say-self-love/

First, let us begin by flipping the script. Self-love comes from within and if you do not love yourself, you cannot expect to fully receive with open arms the love from others so instead of asking why should I love myself, I want you to ask yourself, who needs you to love yourself? In the space below, list 3 people who not only love you but need you to love you and in the column beside their name, you are going to write all the things you love about each person.

As you see from above all the reasons you love your humans, now can you imagine all the reasons they have for loving you.

Self-love is a deliberate way to give yourself care and compassion. The most important relationship we will ever have is the one with ourselves, and we. only get one of us and we are with ourselves until the day we die so why not enjoy our company and love who we are? Why not put us first?

From time to time, we all have self doubt and negative thoughts as it is part of our human nature. There are times when I catch myself participating in negative self-talk and what I have said to myself have been things that I would not say to anyone else. Why did I find it acceptable to think and say them about myself? I've learned to acknowledge when I am in that self doubt mode or having negative self talk, but I do not participate in it anymore. I am bigger than that, I know my worth! You will know your worth too by the end of these 6 months (you may already)!

Loving yourself is where true happiness lies. Once you begin to love yourself, things in all areas of your life begin to fall into place. I know this from my own personal experience. Practicing self- love has helped me improve my relationships with my kids, boyfriend, friends, clients, and co-workers. It has been a great motivator to keep working on my goals and to focus on myself and the things that are important to me. Self Love will always be a journey of mine as I believe that as my love of my self grows, I will continue to see and feel the improvements in my life, body, health, and happiness.

I want you to wake up each morning and go through your days and remind yourself how great of a human you are, how you deserve the best things in life, and that you are working on getting to be where you need to be.

Self-love is not working yourself so that you need a spa day, it is looking ahead and schedule care on your days like a doctor's appointment.

Describe a personal situation in which you were self-critical and viewed yourself with negative judgment. Talk about how it made you feel.

Now describe a time when someone told you about a challenging situation. Talk about how you responded. I also want to talk to you about how you may have responded to your person's situation as if it were your own, how would your response differ?

SELF-AWARENESS

According to Google: "conscious knowledge of one's own character, feelings, motives, and desires." Self-understanding can be painful at times, but it is an important key to our growth and maintaining our belief that we are worthy.

Becoming aware does not mean you judge yourself it is more about paying attention to yourself without judgement. There are many benefits to being self-aware, many of which you have complete control over. Some of the benefits are listed below:

Understand yourself better. As you become self-aware, you become more aware of your capabilities, your strengths, and the areas in which you need to work on and then work on those if you wish. This will also help you with your decision-making and acting on impulse.

Increases your happiness. As you become aware of your emotions and thoughts, you are better able to control both with an increased sense of happiness. As you become aware of your capabilities, an increased sense of self-esteem is also a bonus as you feel accomplished, worthy, smart, etc.

Confidence, motivation to follow your dreams. You'll feel more motivated to reach your goals and show the world your full potential. You will know what you want, what you deserve and can decide to reach for the stars or to settle for less.

Mistakes are no longer the worst thing. You'll begin to embrace "mistakes" and use them as tools for growth. You will see that each time you come back from a "mistake" you will be stronger. Having this awareness not only gives you the ability to become an expert of your emotions and behaviours but also the link between them and your thoughts,

Personal relationships in the home and outside. Becoming aware of your strengths and weaknesses within areas such as communication, your emotions, thoughts, etc. will ultimately help you with building your relationships.

Let go of the past. You will realize that your past is just that - your past and can be anything you want it to be. You can perceive your past as a nightmare with abuse and destruction all around you or you can perceive it as fuel that has made you who you are today and with all the not-so-great stuff as strength that helped get you through the rough times.

Imagine everything you have is now gone, all your possessions, relationships, job, and accomplishments/achievements, all gone. Now, ask yourself the following questions: how would it make you feel if you had nothing except for yourself? Can you honestly say that no matter what happens if you truly have nothing but yourself, you will not be affected internally?

ASK YOURSELF:

1. Who am I?

_____

2. How do others see and speak about me?

_____

3. What abilities do I have? What am I good at?

_____

4. When do I truly feel the most like myself?

_____

5 What do I wish people knew about me?

_____

It's time to look at what is not so great or easy about being you. Ask yourself these questions: **(REMEMBER NOT JUDGING whether good or bad)**

1. Where do I struggle most? Where do I need to improve? Remember no judgement

_____

2. What fears hold me back? What habitual emotions hurt me? (we get so used to feeling a certain way in certain situations that it just becomes a habit to feel that way)

_____

3. What do I wish people knew about me that may not be the best thing about me?

_____

As you become more aware about yourself, you'll find you are more proactive than reactive because you are taking the time to acknowledge your thoughts and connect them to your emotions which is what will ultimately create your result. You will notice little things like what sets you off, what makes you question things, your thought process etc.

AWARENESS IS THE FIRST STEP TOWARD GROWTH SO DO NOT JUDGE YOUR THOUGHTS OR TAKE ACTION IN CHANGING THEM RIGHT AWAY. RATHER, PRACTICE BEING COMPASSIONATE TOWARDS YOUR THOUGHTS

STEP ONE TASK: Take time out of your day to be alone, in a quiet, safe space to reflect on your thoughts, emotions, behaviours, and interactions with others you had throughout the day.

STEP TWO: Practice self awareness. As you go through your day, notice how you interact with others. Notice how you feel inside and what comes easy to you and what you struggle with. Work on leaving the judgment out–simply see. When it gets hard to see these things, stop and take 10 deep breaths. Remind yourself that self-awareness is courageous that leads you to a stronger sense of self-worth and purpose. At the end of the day, write down what you have discovered.

TASK: It is great to have multiple sets of eyes on you to really become aware of who you are. I recommend that you begin to seek feedback from your friends, family, co-workers on how they view you under different circumstances such as stressful situations, joyous occasions etc. Pick those who know you best and will be honest with you. Don't judge what they say or get angry at their honesty as this exercise is to help you grow within your own awareness.

TASK: Becoming aware of oneself is an absolute blessing but awareness about those around you can be hugely beneficial as well. Hell, you can even study those on TV; just pay attention to others, to their tone and language when they are speaking, their emotions, their words, and behaviours. You can learn a lot from observing others and when you relate it back to yourself as well. Each day this week, choose one person in your life or on TV, and observe them. Ask these questions:

TASK: practice self awareness LET'S GATHER ALL THE FACTS ABOUT YOU Start with two lists: "I am," and "I am not." The more you uncover, the more you keep adding to your lists.

I AM	I AM NOT

TASK: Use your Thought Download Journal and ask: can you relate to this statement: "I know you're telling me I am worthy, and I Am Somebody, and I can even tell it to myself because I know, in my head, it should be true. But I just do not feel it.

If so, write out the ways in which you can relate. Complete a thought download to figure out all that you feel and why. Re-read what you have written and really examine it. As you go through your journey you may find things you want to add to either list, come back and add them.

COMPARING OURSELVES WITH OTHERS IS A BIG NO-NO!

Comparing ourselves with others is not a great idea for a few good reasons:

1. When we compare ourselves with others, we tend to look at how inadequate we are, and we lose sight of the fact that we are all equal. It is is difficult to see that when you are busy looking at what they have, and you do not.

2. What we see may not be the whole truth. This means if you want to be like Sally because she always shopping and has such nice expensive beautiful things, what you do not know is that she is extremely depressed because she is has mountains of debt.

3. There will always be someone who does something better than you or has something nicer than you.

4. It steals away joy, happiness, self esteem, self-worth.

Do you believe that some individuals are better or worse than others? If you do, then where do you fit in?

Nobody is better or worse than another, we all are equal! Yes, that is right, the Pope, a criminal and me, we are all equally worthy of one another! We are born worthy and that does not change, my friend. No matter what we do or do not do, we are 100% worthy and loveable and there is nothing that anyone can do or say to change that. Being skinnier, having a hundred friends, the amount of money you have, relationship status, what others think or say about you, changing your career, none of these things will change your worth. Our worth throughout our years does not change. My worth when I was drinking 26er of vodka a day is worth the same as I am now as a sober life coach, owning my own Brand. I may not have seen my worth back then, but it was still there, the only difference is now I know my value and worth.

I find myself comparing myself with others whether it be with respect to appearance or job or just where we each are in our lives. It has just become a habit but now I am catching myself doing it, I recognize it, and then turn it into a positive.

Instead of comparing your appearance with another and making yourself feel bad, Say… "It is awesome that we all are unique and have different physical attributes." Or "She is so beautiful." Appreciate someone's beauty without judging your own!

If you run into someone who is better at you at something you could say "How lucky am I to know someone with such great strengths, especially in the areas where I am lacking, I can learn a lot from them." Or "Wow, he shows me that anything is possible." Or "He is so talented, absolutely inspiring."

If you are someone who compares yourself to other people your age and where they are now compared to yourself, you could say… "Wow, she is very good at what she does, definitely motivates me to put my all into my own shit." Or we all lead different paths in life and my path will go where I want it to and if it is to have those 3 children, that house and job then that is what I will get."

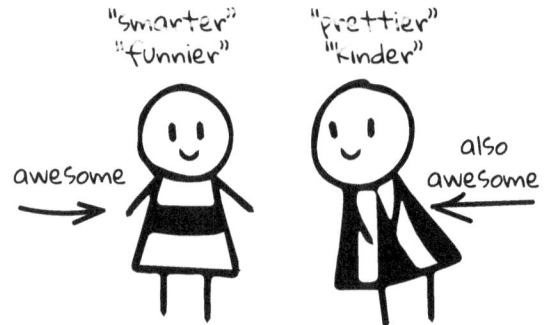

TASK: Be aware of your thoughts. As you hear yourself comparing you to someone else, whether your achievements, appearance, material things, no matter what it is, throughout your days I want you to acknowledge it and ask how you can alter your thinking and turn it into a positive.

Below is a chance for you to practice your skills. I would like you to look back on situations in your life where you know you have compared yourself with others and I want you to acknowledge and ask how you can alter your thinking and turn it into a positive. You can always look back at my examples to see if any fit your situation.

MONTHLY GOALS

DO NOT STOP NOW- YOU ARE ON A ROLL!!:

"Loving ourselves works miracles in our lives" Louise L. Hay

6 MONTHS GOAL	MONTHLY GOAL
GOAL #1	
GOAL #2	

MONTH AT A GLANCE -

STAY TRUE TO YOURSELF

NOTES			

YOU ARE ENOUGH!

Every Sunday review & re-evaluate your goals. Identify obstacles that you faced, along with solutions.

		START CHANGING THE STORY YOU TELL YOURSELF	Say it with me… I AM SOMEBODY

MY WEEK OF AWESOMENESS!
Now that 6 month and monthly goals are done, we now can break down
our goals even further to make them even more achievable

REFLECTIONS OF LAST WEEK:

OBSTACLES I MAY FACE: _____

_____

SOLUTIONS: _____

_____

MY WEEK OF_____

Take 1-5 days this month to go through all your belongings and what you do not use regularly or have multiple of them is time to part with them. When parting with anything that is not actual trash, donate or sell these items.

TIME			

MY WEEK OF AWESOMENESS!

6 Month Goal	6 Month Goal
MONTH	MONTH
WEEK	WEEK
REWARD WHEN I REACH	REWARD WHEN I REACH

MY WEEK OF _____

What time do you want to wake up at, go to bed? How do you want your week to look like?
What events or meetings do you need to attend? Are you planning on having a day of shopping?

AFFIRMATION OF THE DAY: _____

TODAY, I AM LOOKING FORWARD TO

GOALS #1	GOALS #2

HABITS I AM TRACKING	Y/N

THOUGHT DOWNLOAD

TODAY I AM CHOOSING TO FEEL:

C -

T -

F -
A -

R -

I WILL DRINK ___ GLASSES OF WATER TODAY: 1 2 3 4 5 6 7 8 9 10

LOOKING BACK ON MY AMAZINGNESS

MY WINS I CELEBRATE TODAY ARE	TOMORROW I WILL IMPROVE ON

3 THINGS I AM THANKFUL FOR LAST 24 HOURS:

1. ______________________________

2. ______________________________

3. ______________________________

THOUGHT DOWNLOAD

NOTES

AFFIRMATION OF THE DAY: _____

TODAY, I AM LOOKING FORWARD TO

GOALS #1	GOALS #2	HABITS I AM TRACKING	Y/N

THOUGHT DOWNLOAD

TODAY I AM CHOOSING TO FEEL:

C -

T -

F -
A -

R -

I WILL DRINK ____ GLASSES OF WATER TODAY: 1 2 3 4 5 6 7 8 9 10

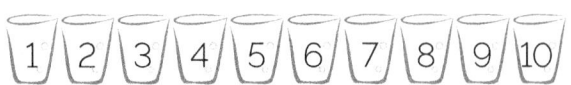

LOOKING BACK ON MY AMAZINGNESS

MY WINS I CELEBRATE TODAY ARE	TOMORROW I WILL IMPROVE ON

3 THINGS I AM THANKFUL FOR LAST 24 HOURS:

1. ____
2. ____
3. ____

THOUGHT DOWNLOAD

NOTES

AFFIRMATION OF THE DAY: _____

TODAY, I AM LOOKING FORWARD TO

GOALS #1	GOALS #2	HABITS I AM TRACKING	Y/N

THOUGHT DOWNLOAD

TODAY I AM CHOOSING TO FEEL:

C -

T -

F -
A -

R -

I WILL DRINK ____ GLASSES OF WATER TODAY: 1 2 3 4 5 6 7 8 9 10

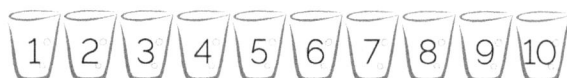

LOOKING BACK ON MY AMAZINGNESS

MY WINS I CELEBRATE TODAY ARE	TOMORROW I WILL IMPROVE ON

3 THINGS I AM THANKFUL FOR LAST 24 HOURS:

1. ______________________________

2. ______________________________

3. ______________________________

THOUGHT DOWNLOAD

NOTES

AFFIRMATION OF THE DAY: --

TODAY, I AM LOOKING FORWARD TO

GOALS #1	GOALS #2

HABITS I AM TRACKING	Y/N

THOUGHT DOWNLOAD

TODAY I AM CHOOSING TO FEEL:

C -

T -

F -
A -

R -

I WILL DRINK ___ GLASSES OF WATER TODAY: 1 2 3 4 5 6 7 8 9 10

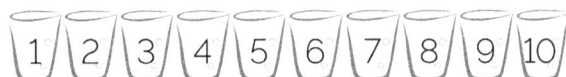

LOOKING BACK ON MY AMAZINGNESS

MY WINS I CELEBRATE TODAY ARE	TOMORROW I WILL IMPROVE ON

3 THINGS I AM THANKFUL FOR LAST 24 HOURS:

1. ______________________________

2. ______________________________

3. ______________________________

THOUGHT DOWNLOAD

NOTES

I AM WHOLE!

AFFIRMATION OF THE DAY: _____

TODAY, I AM LOOKING FORWARD TO

GOALS #1	GOALS #2	HABITS I AM TRACKING	Y/N

THOUGHT DOWNLOAD

TODAY I AM CHOOSING TO FEEL:

C -

T -

F -
A -

R -

I WILL DRINK ___ GLASSES OF WATER TODAY: 1 2 3 4 5 6 7 8 9 10

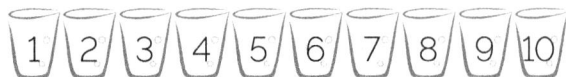

LOOKING BACK ON MY AMAZINGNESS

MY WINS I CELEBRATE TODAY ARE	TOMORROW I WILL IMPROVE ON

3 THINGS I AM THANKFUL FOR LAST 24 HOURS:

1. ______________________________

2. ______________________________

3. ______________________________

THOUGHT DOWNLOAD

NOTES

AFFIRMATION OF THE DAY: _____

TODAY, I AM LOOKING FORWARD TO

GOALS #1	GOALS #2

HABITS I AM TRACKING	Y/N

THOUGHT DOWNLOAD

TODAY I AM CHOOSING TO FEEL:

C -

T -

F -
A -

R -

I WILL DRINK ___ GLASSES OF WATER TODAY: 1 2 3 4 5 6 7 8 9 10

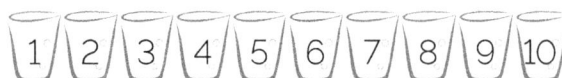

LOOKING BACK ON MY AMAZINGNESS

MY WINS I CELEBRATE TODAY ARE	TOMORROW I WILL IMPROVE ON

3 THINGS I AM THANKFUL FOR LAST 24 HOURS:

1. ______________________________

2. ______________________________

3. ______________________________

THOUGHT DOWNLOAD

NOTES

AFFIRMATION OF THE DAY: _____

TODAY, I AM LOOKING FORWARD TO

GOALS #1	GOALS #2

HABITS I AM TRACKING	Y/N

THOUGHT DOWNLOAD

TODAY I AM CHOOSING TO FEEL:

C -

T -

F -
A -

R -

I WILL DRINK ___ GLASSES OF WATER TODAY: 1 2 3 4 5 6 7 8 9 10

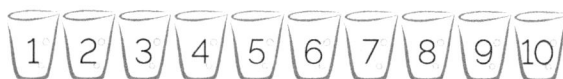

MY WINS I CELEBRATE TODAY ARE	TOMORROW I WILL IMPROVE ON

3 THINGS I AM THANKFUL FOR LAST 24 HOURS:

1. _____

2. _____

3. _____

THOUGHT DOWNLOAD

NOTES

MY WEEK OF AWESOMENESS!
Now that 6 month and monthly goals are done, we now can break down
our goals even further to make them even more achievable

REFLECTIONS OF LAST WEEK:

OBSTACLES I MAY FACE: _____

_____

SOLUTIONS: _____

_____

MY WEEK OF_____

Take **1-5 days** this month to go through all your belongings and what you do not use regularly or have multiple of them is time to part with them. When parting with anything that is not actual trash, donate or sell these items.

TIME			

JENNIFER BULBROOK

MY WEEK OF AWESOMENESS!

6 Month Goal	6 Month Goal
MONTH	MONTH
WEEK	WEEK
REWARD WHEN I REACH	REWARD WHEN I REACH

MY WEEK OF_____
What time do you want to wake up at, go to bed? How do you want your week to look like?
What events or meetings do you need to attend? Are you planning on having a day of shopping?

AFFIRMATION OF THE DAY: _____

TODAY, I AM LOOKING FORWARD TO

GOALS #1	GOALS #2	HABITS I AM TRACKING	Y/N

THOUGHT DOWNLOAD

TODAY I AM CHOOSING TO FEEL:

C -

T -

F -
A -

R -

I WILL DRINK ___ GLASSES OF WATER TODAY: 1 2 3 4 5 6 7 8 9 10

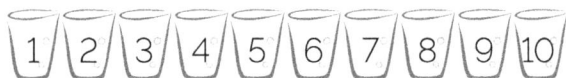

LOOKING BACK ON MY AMAZINGNESS

MY WINS I CELEBRATE TODAY ARE	TOMORROW I WILL IMPROVE ON

3 THINGS I AM THANKFUL FOR LAST 24 HOURS:

1. _____

2. _____

3. _____

THOUGHT DOWNLOAD

NOTES

AFFIRMATION OF THE DAY: _____

TODAY, I AM LOOKING FORWARD TO

GOALS #1	GOALS #2	HABITS I AM TRACKING	Y/N

THOUGHT DOWNLOAD

TODAY I AM CHOOSING TO FEEL:

C -

T -

F -
A -

R -

I WILL DRINK ____ GLASSES OF WATER TODAY: 1 2 3 4 5 6 7 8 9 10

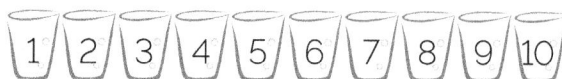

LOOKING BACK ON MY AMAZINGNESS

MY WINS I CELEBRATE TODAY ARE	TOMORROW I WILL IMPROVE ON

3 THINGS I AM THANKFUL FOR LAST 24 HOURS:

1. ______________________________

2. ______________________________

3. ______________________________

THOUGHT DOWNLOAD

NOTES

AFFIRMATION OF THE DAY: _____

TODAY, I AM LOOKING FORWARD TO

GOALS #1	GOALS #2	HABITS I AM TRACKING	Y/N

THOUGHT DOWNLOAD

TODAY I AM CHOOSING TO FEEL:

C -

T -

F -
A -

R -

I WILL DRINK ____ GLASSES OF WATER TODAY: 1 2 3 4 5 6 7 8 9 10

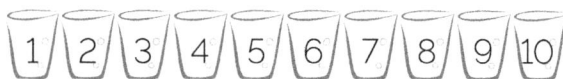

LOOKING BACK ON MY AMAZINGNESS

MY WINS I CELEBRATE TODAY ARE	TOMORROW I WILL IMPROVE ON

3 THINGS I AM THANKFUL FOR LAST 24 HOURS:

1. ____________________
2. ____________________
3. ____________________

THOUGHT DOWNLOAD

NOTES

AFFIRMATION OF THE DAY: _____

TODAY, I AM LOOKING FORWARD TO

GOALS #1	GOALS #2	HABITS I AM TRACKING	Y/N

THOUGHT DOWNLOAD

TODAY I AM CHOOSING TO FEEL:

C -

T -

F -
A -

R -

I WILL DRINK ___ GLASSES OF WATER TODAY: 1 2 3 4 5 6 7 8 9 10

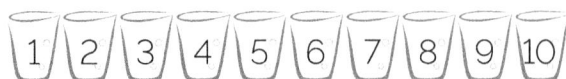

JENNIFER BULBROOK

LOOKING BACK ON MY AMAZINGNESS

MY WINS I CELEBRATE TODAY ARE	TOMORROW I WILL IMPROVE ON

3 THINGS I AM THANKFUL FOR LAST 24 HOURS:

1. ______________________________

2. ______________________________

3. ______________________________

THOUGHT DOWNLOAD

NOTES

AFFIRMATION OF THE DAY: _____

TODAY, I AM LOOKING FORWARD TO

GOALS #1

GOALS #2

HABITS I AM TRACKING	Y/N

THOUGHT DOWNLOAD

TODAY I AM CHOOSING TO FEEL:

C -

T -

F -
A -

R -

I WILL DRINK ___ GLASSES OF WATER TODAY: 1 2 3 4 5 6 7 8 9 10

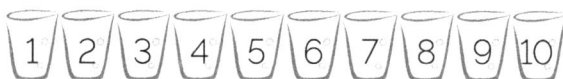

LOOKING BACK ON MY AMAZINGNESS

MY WINS I CELEBRATE TODAY ARE	TOMORROW I WILL IMPROVE ON

3 THINGS I AM THANKFUL FOR LAST 24 HOURS:

1. ______________________________

2. ______________________________

3. ______________________________

THOUGHT DOWNLOAD

NOTES

AFFIRMATION OF THE DAY: _____

TODAY, I AM LOOKING FORWARD TO

GOALS #1	GOALS #2

HABITS I AM TRACKING	Y/N

THOUGHT DOWNLOAD

TODAY I AM CHOOSING TO FEEL:

C -

T -

F -
A -

R -

I WILL DRINK ____ GLASSES OF WATER TODAY: 1 2 3 4 5 6 7 8 9 10

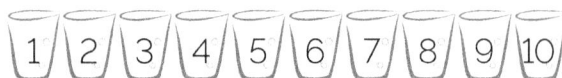

LOOKING BACK ON MY AMAZINGNESS

MY WINS I CELEBRATE TODAY ARE	TOMORROW I WILL IMPROVE ON

3 THINGS I AM THANKFUL FOR LAST 24 HOURS:

1. ____________________

2. ____________________

3. ____________________

THOUGHT DOWNLOAD

NOTES

AFFIRMATION OF THE DAY: _____

TODAY, I AM LOOKING FORWARD TO

GOALS #1	GOALS #2	HABITS I AM TRACKING	Y/N

THOUGHT DOWNLOAD

TODAY I AM CHOOSING TO FEEL:

C -

T -

F -
A -

R -

I WILL DRINK ___ GLASSES OF WATER TODAY: 1 2 3 4 5 6 7 8 9 10

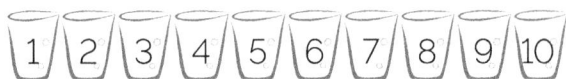

MY WINS I CELEBRATE TODAY ARE	TOMORROW I WILL IMPROVE ON

3 THINGS I AM THANKFUL FOR LAST 24 HOURS:

1. _____

2. _____

3. _____

THOUGHT DOWNLOAD

NOTES

MY WEEK OF AWESOMENESS!
Now that 6 month and monthly goals are done, we now can break down
our goals even further to make them even more achievable

REFLECTIONS OF LAST WEEK:

OBSTACLES I MAY FACE: _____

_____

SOLUTIONS: _____

_____

MY WEEK OF_____
Take 1-5 days this month to go through all your belongings and what you do not use regularly or have multiple of them is time to part with them. When parting with anything that is not actual trash, donate or sell these items.

TIME			

JENNIFER BULBROOK

MY WEEK OF AWESOMENESS!

6 Month Goal	6 Month Goal
MONTH	MONTH
WEEK	WEEK
REWARD WHEN I REACH	REWARD WHEN I REACH

MY WEEK OF_____
What time do you want to wake up at, go to bed? How do you want your week to look like?
What events or meetings do you need to attend? Are you planning on having a day of shopping?

AFFIRMATION OF THE DAY: _

TODAY, I AM LOOKING FORWARD TO

GOALS #1

GOALS #2

HABITS I AM TRACKING	Y/N

THOUGHT DOWNLOAD

TODAY I AM CHOOSING TO FEEL:

C -

T -

F -
A -

R -

I WILL DRINK ___ GLASSES OF WATER TODAY: 1 2 3 4 5 6 7 8 9 10

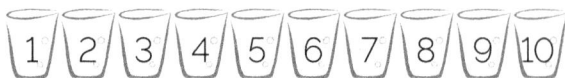

JENNIFER BULBROOK

LOOKING BACK ON MY AMAZINGNESS

MY WINS I CELEBRATE TODAY ARE	TOMORROW I WILL IMPROVE ON

3 THINGS I AM THANKFUL FOR LAST 24 HOURS:

1. ______________________________

2. ______________________________

3. ______________________________

THOUGHT DOWNLOAD

NOTES

AFFIRMATION OF THE DAY: _____

TODAY, I AM LOOKING FORWARD TO

GOALS #1	GOALS #2	HABITS I AM TRACKING	Y/N

THOUGHT DOWNLOAD

TODAY I AM CHOOSING TO FEEL:

C -

T -

F -

A -

R -

I WILL DRINK ___ GLASSES OF WATER TODAY: 1 2 3 4 5 6 7 8 9 10

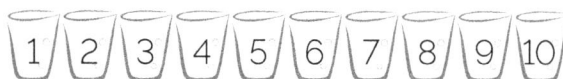

LOOKING BACK ON MY AMAZINGNESS

MY WINS I CELEBRATE TODAY ARE	TOMORROW I WILL IMPROVE ON

3 THINGS I AM THANKFUL FOR LAST 24 HOURS:

1. _____

2. _____

3. _____

THOUGHT DOWNLOAD

NOTES

AFFIRMATION OF THE DAY: _____

TODAY, I AM LOOKING FORWARD TO

GOALS #1	GOALS #2	HABITS I AM TRACKING	Y/N

THOUGHT DOWNLOAD

TODAY I AM CHOOSING TO FEEL:

C -

T -

F -
A -

R -

I WILL DRINK ___ GLASSES OF WATER TODAY: 1 2 3 4 5 6 7 8 9 10

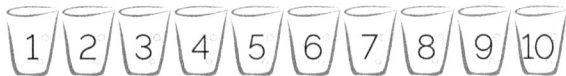

LOOKING BACK ON MY AMAZINGNESS

MY WINS I CELEBRATE TODAY ARE	TOMORROW I WILL IMPROVE ON

3 THINGS I AM THANKFUL FOR LAST 24 HOURS:

1. ____

2. ____

3. ____

THOUGHT DOWNLOAD

NOTES

AFFIRMATION OF THE DAY: _____

TODAY, I AM LOOKING FORWARD TO

GOALS #1	GOALS #2

HABITS I AM TRACKING	Y/N

THOUGHT DOWNLOAD

TODAY I AM CHOOSING TO FEEL:

C -

T -

F -
A -

R -

I WILL DRINK ____ GLASSES OF WATER TODAY: 1 2 3 4 5 6 7 8 9 10

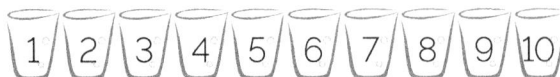

JENNIFER BULBROOK

LOOKING BACK ON MY AMAZINGNESS

MY WINS I CELEBRATE TODAY ARE	TOMORROW I WILL IMPROVE ON

3 THINGS I AM THANKFUL FOR LAST 24 HOURS:

1. ____________________

2. ____________________

3. ____________________

THOUGHT DOWNLOAD

NOTES

AFFIRMATION OF THE DAY: _____

TODAY, I AM LOOKING FORWARD TO

GOALS #1	GOALS #2	HABITS I AM TRACKING	Y/N

THOUGHT DOWNLOAD

TODAY I AM CHOOSING TO FEEL:

C -

T -

F -
A -

R -

I WILL DRINK ___ GLASSES OF WATER TODAY: 1 2 3 4 5 6 7 8 9 10

LOOKING BACK ON MY AMAZINGNESS

MY WINS I CELEBRATE TODAY ARE	TOMORROW I WILL IMPROVE ON

3 THINGS I AM THANKFUL FOR LAST 24 HOURS:

1. ______________________________

2. ______________________________

3. ______________________________

THOUGHT DOWNLOAD

NOTES

AFFIRMATION OF THE DAY: _____

TODAY, I AM LOOKING FORWARD TO

GOALS #1	GOALS #2	HABITS I AM TRACKING	Y/N

THOUGHT DOWNLOAD

TODAY I AM CHOOSING TO FEEL:

C -

T -

F -
A -

R -

I WILL DRINK ____ GLASSES OF WATER TODAY: 1 2 3 4 5 6 7 8 9 10

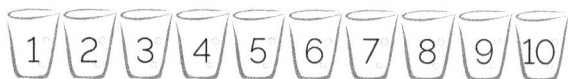

JENNIFER BULBROOK

LOOKING BACK ON MY AMAZINGNESS

MY WINS I CELEBRATE TODAY ARE	TOMORROW I WILL IMPROVE ON

3 THINGS I AM THANKFUL FOR LAST 24 HOURS:

1. ____________________

2. ____________________

3. ____________________

THOUGHT DOWNLOAD

NOTES

AFFIRMATION OF THE DAY: _____

TODAY, I AM LOOKING FORWARD TO

GOALS #1	GOALS #2	HABITS I AM TRACKING	Y/N

THOUGHT DOWNLOAD

TODAY I AM CHOOSING TO FEEL:

C -

T -

F -
A -

R -

I WILL DRINK ___ GLASSES OF WATER TODAY: 1 2 3 4 5 6 7 8 9 10

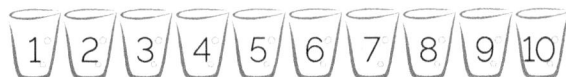

LOOKING BACK ON MY AMAZINGNESS

MY WINS I CELEBRATE TODAY ARE	TOMORROW I WILL IMPROVE ON

3 THINGS I AM THANKFUL FOR LAST 24 HOURS:

1. --

2. --

3. --

THOUGHT DOWNLOAD

NOTES

MY WEEK OF AWESOMENESS!
Now that 6 month and monthly goals are done, we now can break down
our goals even further to make them even more achievable

REFLECTIONS OF LAST WEEK:

OBSTACLES I MAY FACE: _____

_____

SOLUTIONS: _____

_____

MY WEEK OF_____
Take 1-5 days this month to go through all your belongings and what you do not use regularly or have multiple of
them is time to part with them. When parting with anything that is not actual trash, donate or sell these items.

TIME			

MY WEEK OF AWESOMENESS!

6 Month Goal	6 Month Goal
MONTH	MONTH
WEEK	WEEK
REWARD WHEN I REACH	REWARD WHEN I REACH

MY WEEK OF_____

What time do you want to wake up at, go to bed? How do you want your week to look like?
What events or meetings do you need to attend? Are you planning on having a day of shopping?

AFFIRMATION OF THE DAY: _____

TODAY, I AM LOOKING FORWARD TO

GOALS #1	GOALS #2	HABITS I AM TRACKING	Y/N

THOUGHT DOWNLOAD

TODAY I AM CHOOSING TO FEEL:

C -

T -

F -
A -

R -

I WILL DRINK ___ GLASSES OF WATER TODAY: 1 2 3 4 5 6 7 8 9 10

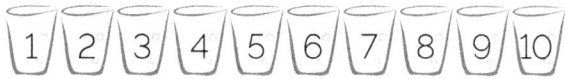

LOOKING BACK ON MY AMAZINGNESS

MY WINS I CELEBRATE TODAY ARE	TOMORROW I WILL IMPROVE ON

3 THINGS I AM THANKFUL FOR LAST 24 HOURS:

1. ______________________________

2. ______________________________

3. ______________________________

THOUGHT DOWNLOAD

NOTES

AFFIRMATION OF THE DAY: --

TODAY, I AM LOOKING FORWARD TO

GOALS #1	GOALS #2	HABITS I AM TRACKING	Y/N

THOUGHT DOWNLOAD

TODAY I AM CHOOSING TO FEEL:

C -

T -

F -
A -

R -

I WILL DRINK ____ GLASSES OF WATER TODAY: 1 2 3 4 5 6 7 8 9 10

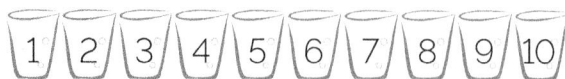

LOOKING BACK ON MY AMAZINGNESS

MY WINS I CELEBRATE TODAY ARE	TOMORROW I WILL IMPROVE ON

3 THINGS I AM THANKFUL FOR LAST 24 HOURS:

1. ____________________
2. ____________________
3. ____________________

THOUGHT DOWNLOAD

NOTES

I AM HEALING!

AFFIRMATION OF THE DAY: _____

TODAY, I AM LOOKING FORWARD TO

GOALS #1 | GOALS #2

HABITS I AM TRACKING	Y/N

THOUGHT DOWNLOAD

TODAY I AM CHOOSING TO FEEL:

C -

T -

F -
A -

R -

I WILL DRINK ___ GLASSES OF WATER TODAY: 1 2 3 4 5 6 7 8 9 10

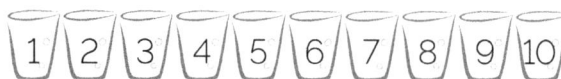

LOOKING BACK ON MY AMAZINGNESS

MY WINS I CELEBRATE TODAY ARE	TOMORROW I WILL IMPROVE ON

3 THINGS I AM THANKFUL FOR LAST 24 HOURS:

1. ______________________________

2. ______________________________

3. ______________________________

THOUGHT DOWNLOAD

NOTES

I LOVE MYSELF UNCODITIONALLY!

AFFIRMATION OF THE DAY: _____

TODAY, I AM LOOKING FORWARD TO

GOALS #1	GOALS #2	HABITS I AM TRACKING	Y/N

THOUGHT DOWNLOAD

TODAY I AM CHOOSING TO FEEL:

C -

T -

F -
A -

R -

I WILL DRINK ___ GLASSES OF WATER TODAY: 1 2 3 4 5 6 7 8 9 10

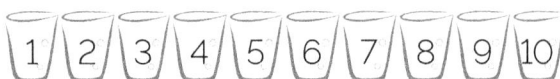

LOOKING BACK ON MY AMAZINGNESS

MY WINS I CELEBRATE TODAY ARE	TOMORROW I WILL IMPROVE ON

3 THINGS I AM THANKFUL FOR LAST 24 HOURS:

1. ______________________________

2. ______________________________

3. ______________________________

THOUGHT DOWNLOAD

NOTES

AFFIRMATION OF THE DAY: _____

TODAY, I AM LOOKING FORWARD TO

GOALS #1	GOALS #2	HABITS I AM TRACKING	Y/N

THOUGHT DOWNLOAD

TODAY I AM CHOOSING TO FEEL:

C -

T -

F -
A -

R -

I WILL DRINK ___ GLASSES OF WATER TODAY: 1 2 3 4 5 6 7 8 9 10

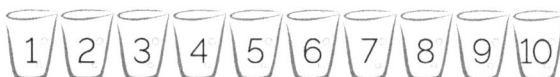

LOOKING BACK ON MY AMAZINGNESS

MY WINS I CELEBRATE TODAY ARE	TOMORROW I WILL IMPROVE ON

3 THINGS I AM THANKFUL FOR LAST 24 HOURS:

1. ______________________________
2. ______________________________
3. ______________________________

THOUGHT DOWNLOAD

NOTES

AFFIRMATION OF THE DAY: _____

TODAY, I AM LOOKING FORWARD TO

GOALS #1	GOALS #2	HABITS I AM TRACKING	Y/N

THOUGHT DOWNLOAD

TODAY I AM CHOOSING TO FEEL:

C -

T -

F -
A -

R -

I WILL DRINK ___ GLASSES OF WATER TODAY: 1 2 3 4 5 6 7 8 9 10

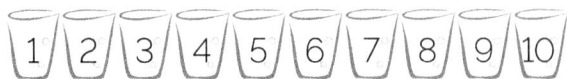

LOOKING BACK ON MY AMAZINGNESS

MY WINS I CELEBRATE TODAY ARE	TOMORROW I WILL IMPROVE ON

3 THINGS I AM THANKFUL FOR LAST 24 HOURS:

1. ______________________________

2. ______________________________

3. ______________________________

THOUGHT DOWNLOAD

NOTES

AFFIRMATION OF THE DAY: _____

TODAY, I AM LOOKING FORWARD TO

GOALS #1	GOALS #2

HABITS I AM TRACKING	Y/N

THOUGHT DOWNLOAD

TODAY I AM CHOOSING TO FEEL:

C -

T -

F -
A -

R -

I WILL DRINK ___ GLASSES OF WATER TODAY: 1 2 3 4 5 6 7 8 9 10

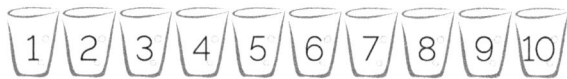

MY WINS I CELEBRATE TODAY ARE	TOMORROW I WILL IMPROVE ON

3 THINGS I AM THANKFUL FOR LAST 24 HOURS:

1. _____

2. _____

3. _____

THOUGHT DOWNLOAD

NOTES

MY WEEK OF AWESOMENESS!
Now that 6 month and monthly goals are done, we now can break down
our goals even further to make them even more achievable

REFLECTIONS OF LAST WEEK:

OBSTACLES I MAY FACE: _____

_____

SOLUTIONS: _____

_____

MY WEEK OF_____
Take 1-5 days this month to go through all your belongings and what you do not use regularly or have multiple of
them is time to part with them. When parting with anything that is not actual trash, donate or sell these items.

TIME			

MY WEEK OF AWESOMENESS!

6 Month Goal	6 Month Goal
MONTH	MONTH
WEEK	WEEK
REWARD WHEN I REACH	REWARD WHEN I REACH

MY WEEK OF_____

What time do you want to wake up at, go to bed? How do you want your week to look like?
What events or meetings do you need to attend? Are you planning on having a day of shopping?

AFFIRMATION OF THE DAY: _____

TODAY, I AM LOOKING FORWARD TO

GOALS #1	GOALS #2

HABITS I AM TRACKING	Y/N

THOUGHT DOWNLOAD

TODAY I AM CHOOSING TO FEEL:

C -

T -

F -
A -

R -

I WILL DRINK ___ GLASSES OF WATER TODAY: 1 2 3 4 5 6 7 8 9 10

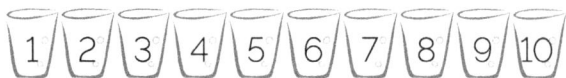

LOOKING BACK ON MY AMAZINGNESS

MY WINS I CELEBRATE TODAY ARE	TOMORROW I WILL IMPROVE ON

3 THINGS I AM THANKFUL FOR LAST 24 HOURS:

1. ______________________________

2. ______________________________

3. ______________________________

THOUGHT DOWNLOAD

NOTES

AFFIRMATION OF THE DAY: _____

TODAY, I AM LOOKING FORWARD TO

GOALS #1	GOALS #2	HABITS I AM TRACKING	Y/N

THOUGHT DOWNLOAD

TODAY I AM CHOOSING TO FEEL:

C -

T -

F -
A -

R -

I WILL DRINK ___ GLASSES OF WATER TODAY: 1 2 3 4 5 6 7 8 9 10

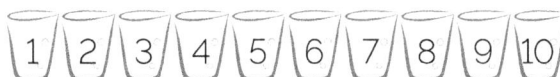

LOOKING BACK ON MY AMAZINGNESS

MY WINS I CELEBRATE TODAY ARE	TOMORROW I WILL IMPROVE ON

3 THINGS I AM THANKFUL FOR LAST 24 HOURS:

1. ______________________________

2. ______________________________

3. ______________________________

THOUGHT DOWNLOAD

NOTES

AFFIRMATION OF THE DAY: _____

TODAY, I AM LOOKING FORWARD TO

GOALS #1	GOALS #2	HABITS I AM TRACKING	Y/N

THOUGHT DOWNLOAD

TODAY I AM CHOOSING TO FEEL:

C -

T -

F -
A -

R -

I WILL DRINK ___ GLASSES OF WATER TODAY: 1 2 3 4 5 6 7 8 9 10

MY WINS I CELEBRATE TODAY ARE	TOMORROW I WILL IMPROVE ON

3 THINGS I AM THANKFUL FOR LAST 24 HOURS:

1. --

2. --

3. --

THOUGHT DOWNLOAD

NOTES

I DESERVE TRUE HAPPINESS!

AFFIRMATION OF THE DAY: _____

TODAY, I AM LOOKING FORWARD TO

GOALS #1	GOALS #2	HABITS I AM TRACKING	Y/N

THOUGHT DOWNLOAD

TODAY I AM CHOOSING TO FEEL:

C -

T -

F -
A -

R -

I WILL DRINK ____ GLASSES OF WATER TODAY: 1 2 3 4 5 6 7 8 9 10

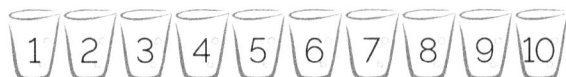

JENNIFER BULBROOK

LOOKING BACK ON MY AMAZINGNESS

MY WINS I CELEBRATE TODAY ARE	TOMORROW I WILL IMPROVE ON

3 THINGS I AM THANKFUL FOR LAST 24 HOURS:

1. ______________________________

2. ______________________________

3. ______________________________

THOUGHT DOWNLOAD

NOTES

AFFIRMATION OF THE DAY: _

TODAY, I AM LOOKING FORWARD TO

GOALS #1 | GOALS #2

HABITS I AM TRACKING	Y/N

THOUGHT DOWNLOAD

TODAY I AM CHOOSING TO FEEL:

C -

T -

F -
A -

R -

I WILL DRINK ___ GLASSES OF WATER TODAY: 1 2 3 4 5 6 7 8 9 10

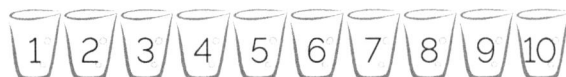

LOOKING BACK ON MY AMAZINGNESS

MY WINS I CELEBRATE TODAY ARE	TOMORROW I WILL IMPROVE ON

3 THINGS I AM THANKFUL FOR LAST 24 HOURS:

1. ______________________________

2. ______________________________

3. ______________________________

THOUGHT DOWNLOAD

NOTES

AFFIRMATION OF THE DAY: _____

TODAY, I AM LOOKING FORWARD TO

GOALS #1	GOALS #2	HABITS I AM TRACKING	Y/N

THOUGHT DOWNLOAD

TODAY I AM CHOOSING TO FEEL:

C -

T -

F -
A -

R -

I WILL DRINK ___ GLASSES OF WATER TODAY: 1 2 3 4 5 6 7 8 9 10

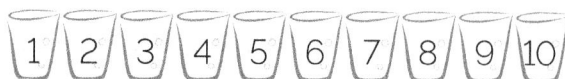

LOOKING BACK ON MY AMAZINGNESS

MY WINS I CELEBRATE TODAY ARE	TOMORROW I WILL IMPROVE ON

3 THINGS I AM THANKFUL FOR LAST 24 HOURS:

1. _____

2. _____

3. _____

THOUGHT DOWNLOAD

NOTES

AFFIRMATION OF THE DAY: _____

TODAY, I AM LOOKING FORWARD TO

GOALS #1	GOALS #2	HABITS I AM TRACKING	Y/N

THOUGHT DOWNLOAD

TODAY I AM CHOOSING TO FEEL:

C -

T -

F -
A -

R -

I WILL DRINK ___ GLASSES OF WATER TODAY: 1 2 3 4 5 6 7 8 9 10

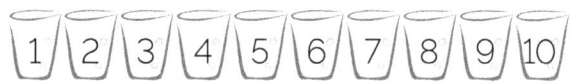

LOOKING BACK ON MY AMAZINGNESS

MY WINS I CELEBRATE TODAY ARE	TOMORROW I WILL IMPROVE ON

3 THINGS I AM THANKFUL FOR LAST 24 HOURS:

1. ______________________________

2. ______________________________

3. ______________________________

THOUGHT DOWNLOAD

NOTES

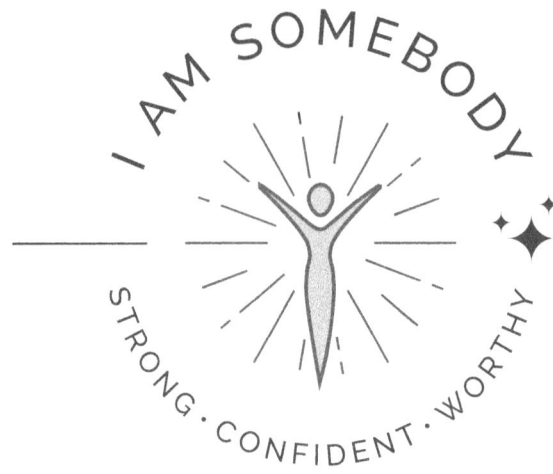

I AM SOMBODY

Transform Your Life Organizer™

Month Four

BUILDING SELF-ACCEPTANCE

The next step in increasing your self-worth is to accept yourself entirely without judgment or excuses by making a commitment to forgive yourself for all that has gone wrong, any struggles, mistakes, bad habits you have, and needs for improvements that you feel you need to make in your life.

Show yourself some compassion, understand that you did your best at that time and didn't have complete control over the situation. Just know your past and your experiences do not define who you are; they do not define your worth.

Talking about our past is not helpful unless we are willing to admit the facts and leave the judgments behind. Admitting what is real about your past is useful but dwelling on it is far from that. In fact, by contrast, it will tear you down. We must understand that our past is over and therefore the story in our minds of our past is the only thing that now exists.

What happened in your past is over and the pain is gone with it, pain does not exist with our past. The pain you are experiencing now is new pain resulting from your current thinking. Your past only defines you depending on how you frame it. We cause our own pain whether past, present, or future...

A little example of a piece of my past. I grew up with a close loving family where there was little yelling. We ate dinner together and took many trips. I earned babysitting money watching my sister when my parents went out. We told each other we loved one another and valued each other's company.

Or

I grew up with a father who was ill and never knew when he was going to die. We went away a lot because my dad would raise money for his work and therefore, I was stuck spending a lot of my time in hotels with other kids. If we were not away, my parents would go out every Friday and Saturday, so I was stuck watching my little sister instead of being able to have fun with my friends.

Now they are both my story, they both are true, it is just how I choose to think and feel about my past that differs. I would rather focus on the positive and be happy than focus on the negative and be sad. So many of us decide to keep our past close to us, we hold it tight as if it were our present and we continue to live it daily.

Do not have any regrets about your past, that does not serve you. Instead, use regret to better your future. If you are working on cutting back on drinking and you then find yourself in the middle of the liquor store aisle, this is when you think about how it will feel if you've already bought the bottle, already drank it and now it is the next day and you are hung over feeling all sorts of nastiness emotionally and physically. Let it help you prevent yourself from going back on your commitment to yourself.

Be mindful, acknowledge your thoughts and feelings, do not just dismiss them. When you begin to feel like you are not worthy, take a minute and explore what thoughts you are thinking. If you must, wait until the feeling passes and then ask yourself the question again. Allow yourself to feel the emotions without judgment. You will eventually see different patterns and connections between certain situations and thought processes/emotions and results and in which you will be able to change as you wish.

Forget about being the perfect human, whether appearance or capabilities, there is no such thing. We all have flaws, there will always be something that someone does not like about us or that we will not love about ourselves. That is life. Our imperfections make us unique while our failures help us grow and become more accepting of ourselves.

Remember You Are Enough and why because, say it with me... I Am Somebody!

These questions will help you better understand how accepting you are, and what might be holding you back from fully accepting who you are as a human.

What is most authentic about you?

Can you think and speak kindly about yourself? Are you non-judgmental towards yourself? Can you give yourself a break? Are you gentle with yourself?

Are you taking care of your needs? Diet, exercise, rest, relaxation, fun, social interaction, alone time – are you giving yourself time for these things?

Do you accept love from others? Do you push love away?

Do you accept love from yourself? Do you push self love away?

Rate your belief in each statement below on a scale from 0 (not at all) to 10 (completely):

1. I believe in myself _____

2. I am just as worthy as other people _____

3. I would rather be me than anyone else _____

4. I am proud of my achievements _____

5. I feel good when I am complimented _____

6. I can handle criticism well _____

7. I believe in my ideas _____

8. I love trying new things _____

9. I respect myself _____

10. I like the way I look _____

11. I love myself even when others reject me _____

12. I know my positive qualities _____

13. I focus on my successes and not my failures _____

14. I am not afraid to make mistakes _____

15. I am happy to be me _____

Add up all the ratings for these 15 statements to get your total score _____

Rate your overall sense of self-esteem on a scale from 0 (I completely dislike who I am) to 10 (I completely love who I am) _____

Next, what would need to change for you to move up one point on the rating scale? (For example, if you rated yourself a 5, what changes need to be made for you to be at a 6?)

Please look at what you wrote for the previous question and brainstorm ways to make those changes happen. If you say that to move up to a 6, you need to lose 50 pounds, now is the time to explore ways to lose 50 pounds and decide on a way to execute the plan. If you say to feel more worthy then you will be able to move up a level, then write what you need to do to increase your self worth, and plan to execute it.

I then want you to review your answers when needed and practice your plans as needed.

INCREASE SELF-LOVE

Now that you have worked on accepting who you are, it's time to begin to build love and care for yourself. Make it a goal to show yourself kindness, compassion, patience, and generosity each day.

Be aware of that little negative voice in your ear, the one that likes to say you are not good enough or smart enough, the one that keeps you from achieving your goals, I call mine, Juicifer (Lucifer but with a J lol). As you begin to hear this voice, ask yourself whether there is any fact to what is being said or if it even needs to be said, if not, then remind yourself that no matter what, YOU ARE WORTHY! Sometimes we are the ones to tell ourselves the ugliest, least loving words that we hear all day, sometimes all week. These stories are often reactive, have lack of evidence for truth, and have been in our minds for as long as we can remember.

TASK: Instead of ignoring or avoiding your negative thoughts, approach them with love and compassion and see what happens when we see ourselves in a different light. Set a timer for two minutes. Under "Lies", will dump all the negative thoughts you have about yourself. Start at your head and go down to your toes; writing down each thing you have heard or thought about you that does not serve you. Then, set a timer for two new minutes. Under "Truths" you will write an "I am…" statement that is an opposite, but TRUTH of the lie you are telling yourself in the first column.

LIES	TRUTHS
I will never be loved for who I am because of my mood swings	I am loveable no matter my mood swings.

If you feel comfortable, make a post, add to your story, and share one or more of your truths with me @ IAM_SOMEBODY_2 share your page. If you are not ready yet, just read your list of "I am…" statements to yourself.

Commit to being more positive and joyful when talking to yourself about yourself, pay attention to the tone you are using. The tone and the wording will make a difference so just be mindful of that. I suggest beginning with these simple statements but if you do not completely believe them then choose three that you do feel fit where you are right now. You must believe what you are thinking or saying your progress will be null.

1. I am special

2. I love myself wholeheartedly or I am learning to love myself wholeheartedly, and

3. I am worthy or I am in the process of learning my true worth

TASK: IN EACH HEART WRITE WHAT YOU LOVE ABOUT YOURSELF. IT CAN BE ANYTHING FROM YOUR EYES TO YOUR PERSONALITY TO WHAT YOU ARE GOOD AT. IF YOU NEED, DRAW MORE HEARTS OR WRITE MORE THAN ONE WORD IN EACH HEART. USE SOME EXTRA PAPER IF NECESSARY.

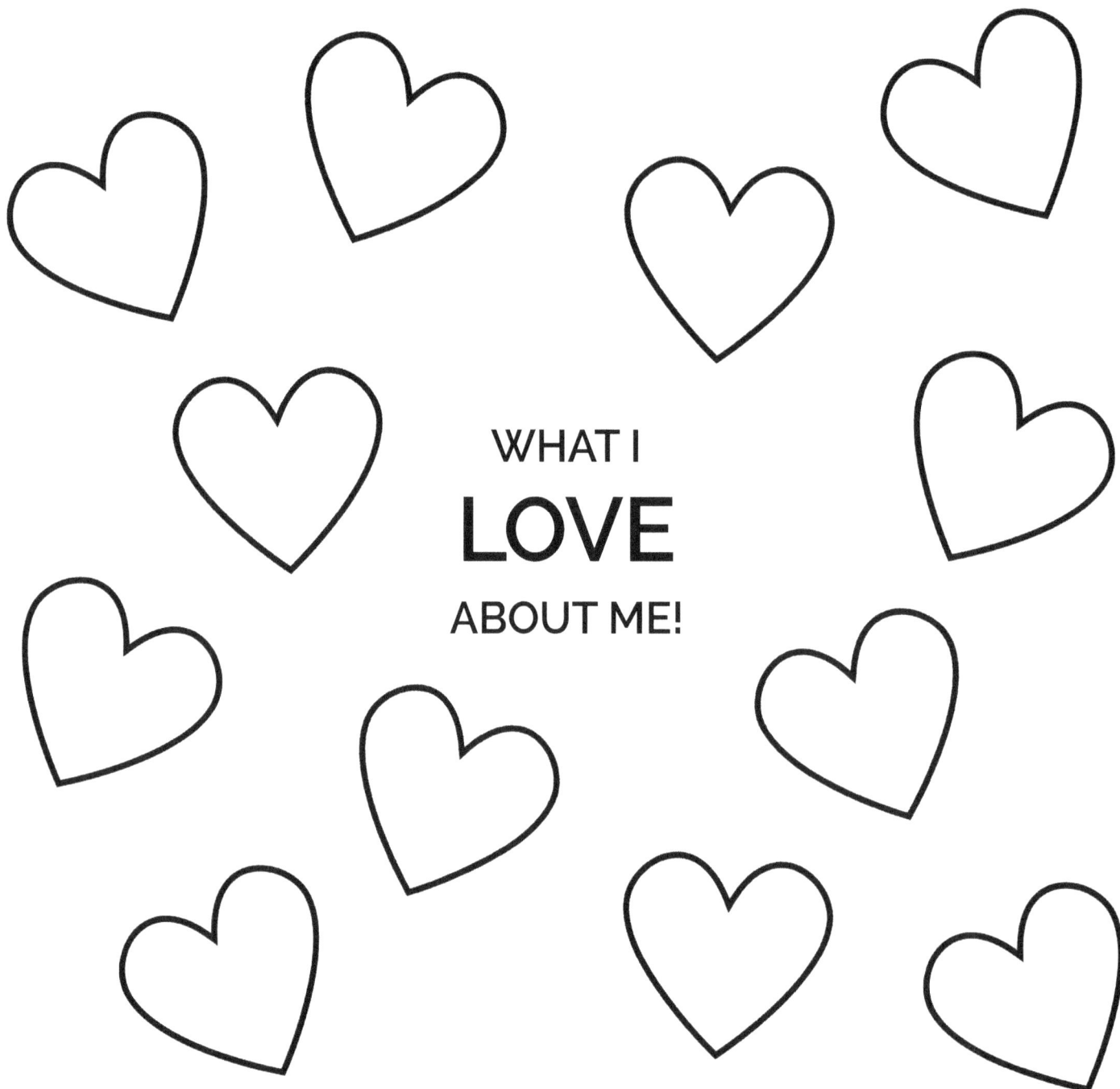

WHAT I
LOVE
ABOUT ME!

MONTHLY GOALS

AND JUST LIKE THAT YOU ARE ONTO ANOTHER MONTH:

"Why should we worry about what others think of us, do we have more confidence in their opinions than we do our own?" Brigham Young

6 MONTHS GOAL	MONTHLY GOAL
GOAL #1	
GOAL #2	

SPEND TIME IN SILENCE

NOTES			

IT IS NEVER TOO LATE TO BE WHO YOU WANT TO BE!

Every Sunday review & re-evaluate your goals. Identify obstacles that you faced, along with solutions.

		YOU BECOME BETTER ACQUAINTED WITH WHO YOU ARE AND WHERE YOU SHOULD BE WHEN YOU SIT IN SILENCE REGULARLY.	Say it with me... I AM SOMEBODY

MY WEEK OF AWESOMENESS!
Now that 6 month and monthly goals are done, we now can break down
our goals even further to make them even more achievable

REFLECTIONS OF LAST WEEK:

OBSTACLES I MAY FACE: _____

_____

SOLUTIONS: _____

_____

MY WEEK OF_____
Take 1-5 days this month to go through all your belongings and what you do not use regularly or have multiple of them is time to part with them. When parting with anything that is not actual trash, donate or sell these items.

TIME			

JENNIFER BULBROOK

MY WEEK OF AWESOMENESS!

6 Month Goal	6 Month Goal
MONTH	MONTH
WEEK	WEEK
REWARD WHEN I REACH	REWARD WHEN I REACH

MY WEEK OF_____
What time do you want to wake up at, go to bed? How do you want your week to look like?
What events or meetings do you need to attend? Are you planning on having a day of shopping?

AFFIRMATION OF THE DAY: _____

TODAY, I AM LOOKING FORWARD TO

GOALS #1	GOALS #2	HABITS I AM TRACKING	Y/N

THOUGHT DOWNLOAD

TODAY I AM CHOOSING TO FEEL:

C -

T -

F -
A -

R -

I WILL DRINK ____ GLASSES OF WATER TODAY: 1 2 3 4 5 6 7 8 9 10

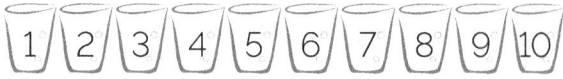

JENNIFER BULBROOK

LOOKING BACK ON MY AMAZINGNESS

MY WINS I CELEBRATE TODAY ARE	TOMORROW I WILL IMPROVE ON

3 THINGS I AM THANKFUL FOR LAST 24 HOURS:

1. ______________________________

2. ______________________________

3. ______________________________

THOUGHT DOWNLOAD

NOTES

AFFIRMATION OF THE DAY: --

TODAY, I AM LOOKING FORWARD TO

GOALS #1	GOALS #2	HABITS I AM TRACKING	Y/N

THOUGHT DOWNLOAD

TODAY I AM CHOOSING TO FEEL:

C -

T -

F -
A -

R -

I WILL DRINK ___ GLASSES OF WATER TODAY: 1 2 3 4 5 6 7 8 9 10

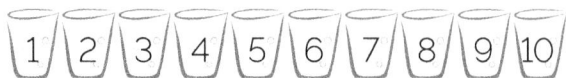

LOOKING BACK ON MY AMAZINGNESS

MY WINS I CELEBRATE TODAY ARE	TOMORROW I WILL IMPROVE ON

3 THINGS I AM THANKFUL FOR LAST 24 HOURS:

1. ______________________________

2. ______________________________

3. ______________________________

THOUGHT DOWNLOAD

NOTES

AFFIRMATION OF THE DAY: _____

TODAY, I AM LOOKING FORWARD TO

GOALS #1	GOALS #2	HABITS I AM TRACKING	Y/N

THOUGHT DOWNLOAD

TODAY I AM CHOOSING TO FEEL:

C -

T -

F -
A -

R -

I WILL DRINK ___ GLASSES OF WATER TODAY: 1 2 3 4 5 6 7 8 9 10

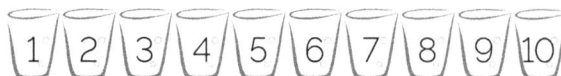

LOOKING BACK ON MY AMAZINGNESS

MY WINS I CELEBRATE TODAY ARE	TOMORROW I WILL IMPROVE ON

3 THINGS I AM THANKFUL FOR LAST 24 HOURS:

1. ____
2. ____
3. ____

THOUGHT DOWNLOAD

NOTES

AFFIRMATION OF THE DAY: _____

TODAY, I AM LOOKING FORWARD TO

GOALS #1	GOALS #2	HABITS I AM TRACKING	Y/N

THOUGHT DOWNLOAD

TODAY I AM CHOOSING TO FEEL:

C -

T -

F -
A -

R -

I WILL DRINK ___ GLASSES OF WATER TODAY: 1 2 3 4 5 6 7 8 9 10

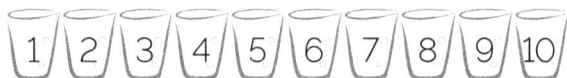

LOOKING BACK ON MY AMAZINGNESS

MY WINS I CELEBRATE TODAY ARE	TOMORROW I WILL IMPROVE ON

3 THINGS I AM THANKFUL FOR LAST 24 HOURS:

1. ______________________________

2. ______________________________

3. ______________________________

THOUGHT DOWNLOAD

NOTES

AFFIRMATION OF THE DAY: _____

TODAY, I AM LOOKING FORWARD TO

GOALS #1	GOALS #2	HABITS I AM TRACKING	Y/N

THOUGHT DOWNLOAD

TODAY I AM CHOOSING TO FEEL:

C -

T -

F -
A -

R -

I WILL DRINK ___ GLASSES OF WATER TODAY: 1 2 3 4 5 6 7 8 9 10

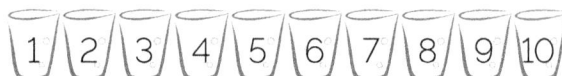

LOOKING BACK ON MY AMAZINGNESS

MY WINS I CELEBRATE TODAY ARE	TOMORROW I WILL IMPROVE ON

3 THINGS I AM THANKFUL FOR LAST 24 HOURS:

1. --

2. --

3. --

THOUGHT DOWNLOAD

NOTES

AFFIRMATION OF THE DAY: --

TODAY, I AM LOOKING FORWARD TO

GOALS #1	GOALS #2	HABITS I AM TRACKING	Y/N

THOUGHT DOWNLOAD

TODAY I AM CHOOSING TO FEEL:

C -

T -

F -
A -

R -

I WILL DRINK ____ GLASSES OF WATER TODAY: 1 2 3 4 5 6 7 8 9 10

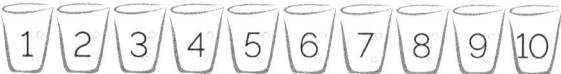

LOOKING BACK ON MY AMAZINGNESS

MY WINS I CELEBRATE TODAY ARE	TOMORROW I WILL IMPROVE ON

3 THINGS I AM THANKFUL FOR LAST 24 HOURS:

1. ______________________________

2. ______________________________

3. ______________________________

THOUGHT DOWNLOAD

NOTES

AFFIRMATION OF THE DAY: _____

TODAY, I AM LOOKING FORWARD TO

GOALS #1	GOALS #2	HABITS I AM TRACKING	Y/N

THOUGHT DOWNLOAD

TODAY I AM CHOOSING TO FEEL:

C -

T -

F -
A -

R -

I WILL DRINK ____ GLASSES OF WATER TODAY: 1 2 3 4 5 6 7 8 9 10

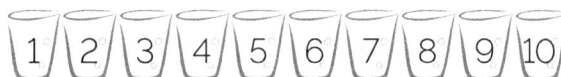

MY WINS I CELEBRATE TODAY ARE	TOMORROW I WILL IMPROVE ON

3 THINGS I AM THANKFUL FOR LAST 24 HOURS:

1. _____

2. _____

3. _____

THOUGHT DOWNLOAD

NOTES

MY WEEK OF AWESOMENESS!
Now that 6 month and monthly goals are done, we now can break down
our goals even further to make them even more achievable

REFLECTIONS OF LAST WEEK:

OBSTACLES I MAY FACE: _____

_____

SOLUTIONS: _____

_____

MY WEEK OF_____
Take 1-5 days this month to go through all your belongings and what you do not use regularly or have multiple of them is time to part with them. When parting with anything that is not actual trash, donate or sell these items.

TIME			

MY WEEK OF AWESOMENESS!

6 Month Goal	6 Month Goal
MONTH	MONTH
WEEK	WEEK
REWARD WHEN I REACH	REWARD WHEN I REACH

MY WEEK OF _____

What time do you want to wake up at, go to bed? How do you want your week to look like?
What events or meetings do you need to attend? Are you planning on having a day of shopping?

AFFIRMATION OF THE DAY: _____

TODAY, I AM LOOKING FORWARD TO

GOALS #1	GOALS #2	HABITS I AM TRACKING	Y/N

THOUGHT DOWNLOAD

TODAY I AM CHOOSING TO FEEL:

C -

T -

F -
A -

R -

I WILL DRINK ____ GLASSES OF WATER TODAY: 1 2 3 4 5 6 7 8 9 10

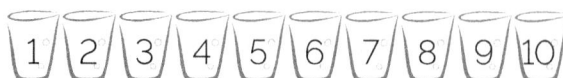

LOOKING BACK ON MY AMAZINGNESS

MY WINS I CELEBRATE TODAY ARE	TOMORROW I WILL IMPROVE ON

3 THINGS I AM THANKFUL FOR LAST 24 HOURS:

1. ______________________________

2. ______________________________

3. ______________________________

THOUGHT DOWNLOAD

NOTES

AFFIRMATION OF THE DAY: _____

TODAY, I AM LOOKING FORWARD TO

GOALS #1	GOALS #2

HABITS I AM TRACKING	Y/N

THOUGHT DOWNLOAD

TODAY I AM CHOOSING TO FEEL:

C -

T -

F -
A -

R -

I WILL DRINK ___ GLASSES OF WATER TODAY: 1 2 3 4 5 6 7 8 9 10

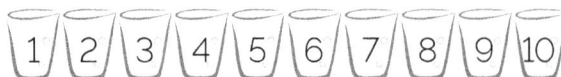

LOOKING BACK ON MY AMAZINGNESS

MY WINS I CELEBRATE TODAY ARE	TOMORROW I WILL IMPROVE ON

3 THINGS I AM THANKFUL FOR LAST 24 HOURS:

1. _____

2. _____

3. _____

THOUGHT DOWNLOAD

NOTES

AFFIRMATION OF THE DAY: _____

TODAY, I AM LOOKING FORWARD TO

GOALS #1	GOALS #2

HABITS I AM TRACKING	Y/N

THOUGHT DOWNLOAD

TODAY I AM CHOOSING TO FEEL:

C -

T -

F -
A -

R -

I WILL DRINK ____ GLASSES OF WATER TODAY: 1 2 3 4 5 6 7 8 9 10

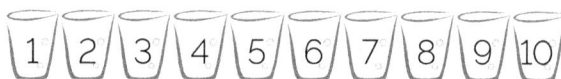

LOOKING BACK ON MY AMAZINGNESS

MY WINS I CELEBRATE TODAY ARE	TOMORROW I WILL IMPROVE ON

3 THINGS I AM THANKFUL FOR LAST 24 HOURS:

1. ______________________________

2. ______________________________

3. ______________________________

THOUGHT DOWNLOAD

NOTES

AFFIRMATION OF THE DAY: _____

TODAY, I AM LOOKING FORWARD TO

GOALS #1	GOALS #2

HABITS I AM TRACKING	Y/N

THOUGHT DOWNLOAD

TODAY I AM CHOOSING TO FEEL:

C -

T -

F -
A -

R -

I WILL DRINK ___ GLASSES OF WATER TODAY: 1 2 3 4 5 6 7 8 9 10

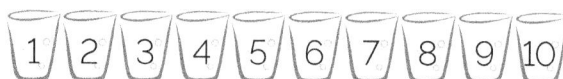

LOOKING BACK ON MY AMAZINGNESS

MY WINS I CELEBRATE TODAY ARE	TOMORROW I WILL IMPROVE ON

3 THINGS I AM THANKFUL FOR LAST 24 HOURS:

1. ______________________________

2. ______________________________

3. ______________________________

THOUGHT DOWNLOAD

NOTES

AFFIRMATION OF THE DAY: _____

TODAY, I AM LOOKING FORWARD TO

GOALS #1	GOALS #2

HABITS I AM TRACKING	Y/N

THOUGHT DOWNLOAD

TODAY I AM CHOOSING TO FEEL:

C -

T -

F -
A -

R -

I WILL DRINK ___ GLASSES OF WATER TODAY: 1 2 3 4 5 6 7 8 9 10

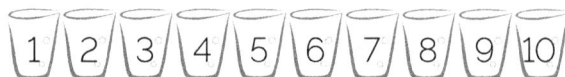

LOOKING BACK ON MY AMAZINGNESS

MY WINS I CELEBRATE TODAY ARE	TOMORROW I WILL IMPROVE ON

3 THINGS I AM THANKFUL FOR LAST 24 HOURS:

1. ______________________________

2. ______________________________

3. ______________________________

THOUGHT DOWNLOAD

NOTES

AFFIRMATION OF THE DAY: _____

TODAY, I AM LOOKING FORWARD TO

GOALS #1	GOALS #2	HABITS I AM TRACKING	Y/N

THOUGHT DOWNLOAD

TODAY I AM CHOOSING TO FEEL:

C -

T -

F -
A -

R -

I WILL DRINK ___ GLASSES OF WATER TODAY: 1 2 3 4 5 6 7 8 9 10

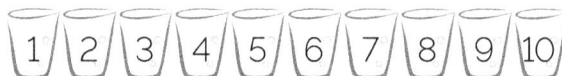

JENNIFER BULBROOK

LOOKING BACK ON MY AMAZINGNESS

MY WINS I CELEBRATE TODAY ARE	TOMORROW I WILL IMPROVE ON

3 THINGS I AM THANKFUL FOR LAST 24 HOURS:

1. _____

2. _____

3. _____

THOUGHT DOWNLOAD

NOTES

AFFIRMATION OF THE DAY: _____

TODAY, I AM LOOKING FORWARD TO

GOALS #1	GOALS #2

HABITS I AM TRACKING	Y/N

THOUGHT DOWNLOAD

TODAY I AM CHOOSING TO FEEL:

C -

T -

F -
A -

R -

I WILL DRINK ___ GLASSES OF WATER TODAY: 1 2 3 4 5 6 7 8 9 10

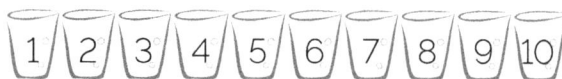

MY WINS I CELEBRATE TODAY ARE	TOMORROW I WILL IMPROVE ON

3 THINGS I AM THANKFUL FOR LAST 24 HOURS:

1. _____

2. _____

3. _____

THOUGHT DOWNLOAD

NOTES

MY WEEK OF AWESOMENESS!
Now that 6 month and monthly goals are done, we now can break down
our goals even further to make them even more achievable

REFLECTIONS OF LAST WEEK:

OBSTACLES I MAY FACE: _____

_____

SOLUTIONS: _____

_____

MY WEEK OF_____
Take 1-5 days this month to go through all your belongings and what you do not use regularly or have multiple of them is time to part with them. When parting with anything that is not actual trash, donate or sell these items.

TIME			

MY WEEK OF AWESOMENESS!

6 Month Goal	6 Month Goal
MONTH	MONTH
WEEK	WEEK
REWARD WHEN I REACH	REWARD WHEN I REACH

MY WEEK OF _____

What time do you want to wake up at, go to bed? How do you want your week to look like?
What events or meetings do you need to attend? Are you planning on having a day of shopping?

AFFIRMATION OF THE DAY: _____

TODAY, I AM LOOKING FORWARD TO

GOALS #1	GOALS #2

HABITS I AM TRACKING	Y/N

THOUGHT DOWNLOAD

TODAY I AM CHOOSING TO FEEL:

C -

T -

F -
A -

R -

I WILL DRINK ___ GLASSES OF WATER TODAY: 1 2 3 4 5 6 7 8 9 10

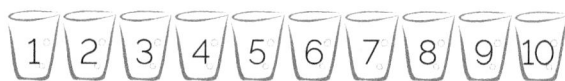

LOOKING BACK ON MY AMAZINGNESS

MY WINS I CELEBRATE TODAY ARE	TOMORROW I WILL IMPROVE ON

3 THINGS I AM THANKFUL FOR LAST 24 HOURS:

1. ______________________________

2. ______________________________

3. ______________________________

THOUGHT DOWNLOAD

NOTES

AFFIRMATION OF THE DAY: _____

TODAY, I AM LOOKING FORWARD TO

GOALS #1	GOALS #2	HABITS I AM TRACKING	Y/N

THOUGHT DOWNLOAD

TODAY I AM CHOOSING TO FEEL:

C -

T -

F -
A -

R -

I WILL DRINK ___ GLASSES OF WATER TODAY: 1 2 3 4 5 6 7 8 9 10

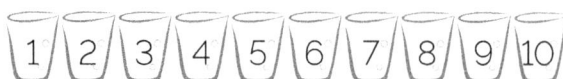

LOOKING BACK ON MY AMAZINGNESS

MY WINS I CELEBRATE TODAY ARE	TOMORROW I WILL IMPROVE ON

3 THINGS I AM THANKFUL FOR LAST 24 HOURS:

1. ______________________________

2. ______________________________

3. ______________________________

THOUGHT DOWNLOAD

NOTES

AFFIRMATION OF THE DAY: _

TODAY, I AM LOOKING FORWARD TO

GOALS #1	GOALS #2	HABITS I AM TRACKING	Y/N

THOUGHT DOWNLOAD

TODAY I AM CHOOSING TO FEEL:

C -

T -

F -
A -

R -

I WILL DRINK ___ GLASSES OF WATER TODAY: 1 2 3 4 5 6 7 8 9 10

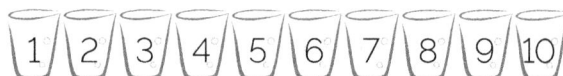

LOOKING BACK ON MY AMAZINGNESS

MY WINS I CELEBRATE TODAY ARE	TOMORROW I WILL IMPROVE ON

3 THINGS I AM THANKFUL FOR LAST 24 HOURS:

1. ______________________________

2. ______________________________

3. ______________________________

THOUGHT DOWNLOAD

NOTES

AFFIRMATION OF THE DAY: _____

TODAY, I AM LOOKING FORWARD TO

GOALS #1	GOALS #2	HABITS I AM TRACKING	Y/N

THOUGHT DOWNLOAD

TODAY I AM CHOOSING TO FEEL:

C -

T -

F -
A -

R -

I WILL DRINK ___ GLASSES OF WATER TODAY: 1 2 3 4 5 6 7 8 9 10

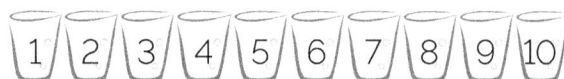

LOOKING BACK ON MY AMAZINGNESS

MY WINS I CELEBRATE TODAY ARE	TOMORROW I WILL IMPROVE ON

3 THINGS I AM THANKFUL FOR LAST 24 HOURS:

1. ______________________________

2. ______________________________

3. ______________________________

THOUGHT DOWNLOAD

NOTES

I WILL DO THIS!

AFFIRMATION OF THE DAY: --

TODAY, I AM LOOKING FORWARD TO

GOALS #1	GOALS #2	HABITS I AM TRACKING	Y/N

THOUGHT DOWNLOAD

TODAY I AM CHOOSING TO FEEL:

C -

T -

F -
A -

R -

I WILL DRINK ___ GLASSES OF WATER TODAY: 1 2 3 4 5 6 7 8 9 10

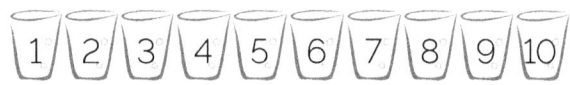

JENNIFER BULBROOK

LOOKING BACK ON MY AMAZINGNESS

MY WINS I CELEBRATE TODAY ARE	TOMORROW I WILL IMPROVE ON

3 THINGS I AM THANKFUL FOR LAST 24 HOURS:

1. ______________________________

2. ______________________________

3. ______________________________

THOUGHT DOWNLOAD

NOTES

AFFIRMATION OF THE DAY: _____

TODAY, I AM LOOKING FORWARD TO

GOALS #1	GOALS #2

HABITS I AM TRACKING	Y/N

THOUGHT DOWNLOAD

TODAY I AM CHOOSING TO FEEL:

C -

T -

F -
A -

R -

I WILL DRINK ___ GLASSES OF WATER TODAY: 1 2 3 4 5 6 7 8 9 10

LOOKING BACK ON MY AMAZINGNESS

MY WINS I CELEBRATE TODAY ARE	TOMORROW I WILL IMPROVE ON

3 THINGS I AM THANKFUL FOR LAST 24 HOURS:

1. ____________________

2. ____________________

3. ____________________

THOUGHT DOWNLOAD

NOTES

AFFIRMATION OF THE DAY: _____

TODAY, I AM LOOKING FORWARD TO

GOALS #1	GOALS #2

HABITS I AM TRACKING	Y/N

THOUGHT DOWNLOAD

TODAY I AM CHOOSING TO FEEL:

C -

T -

F -
A -

R -

I WILL DRINK ____ GLASSES OF WATER TODAY: 1 2 3 4 5 6 7 8 9 10

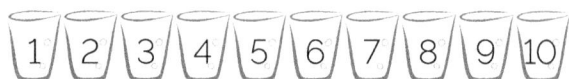

MY WINS I CELEBRATE TODAY ARE	TOMORROW I WILL IMPROVE ON

3 THINGS I AM THANKFUL FOR LAST 24 HOURS:

1. _____

2. _____

3. _____

THOUGHT DOWNLOAD

NOTES

MY WEEK OF AWESOMENESS!
Now that 6 month and monthly goals are done, we now can break down
our goals even further to make them even more achievable

REFLECTIONS OF LAST WEEK:

OBSTACLES I MAY FACE: _____

_____

SOLUTIONS: _____

_____

MY WEEK OF_____
Take 1-5 days this month to go through all your belongings and what you do not use regularly or have multiple of
them is time to part with them. When parting with anything that is not actual trash, donate or sell these items.

TIME			

MY WEEK OF AWESOMENESS!

6 Month Goal	6 Month Goal
MONTH	MONTH
WHEN	WEEK
REWARD WHEN I REACH	REWARD WHEN I REACH

MY WEEK OF_____
What time do you want to wake up at, go to bed? How do you want your week to look like?
What events or meetings do you need to attend? Are you planning on having a day of shopping?

A LITTLE SELF-CARE EVERYDAY GOES A LONG WAY!

AFFIRMATION OF THE DAY: _____

TODAY, I AM LOOKING FORWARD TO

GOALS #1	GOALS #2	HABITS I AM TRACKING	Y/N

THOUGHT DOWNLOAD

TODAY I AM CHOOSING TO FEEL:

C -

T -

F -
A -

R -

I WILL DRINK ___ GLASSES OF WATER TODAY: 1 2 3 4 5 6 7 8 9 10

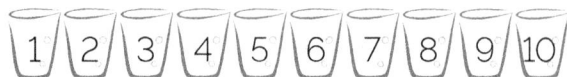

LOOKING BACK ON MY AMAZINGNESS

MY WINS I CELEBRATE TODAY ARE	TOMORROW I WILL IMPROVE ON

3 THINGS I AM THANKFUL FOR LAST 24 HOURS:

1. ______

2. ______

3. ______

THOUGHT DOWNLOAD

NOTES

AFFIRMATION OF THE DAY: _____

TODAY, I AM LOOKING FORWARD TO

GOALS #1	GOALS #2

HABITS I AM TRACKING	Y/N

THOUGHT DOWNLOAD

TODAY I AM CHOOSING TO FEEL:

C -

T -

F -
A -

R -

I WILL DRINK ___ GLASSES OF WATER TODAY: 1 2 3 4 5 6 7 8 9 10

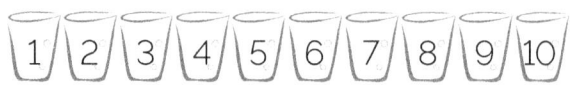

LOOKING BACK ON MY AMAZINGNESS

MY WINS I CELEBRATE TODAY ARE	TOMORROW I WILL IMPROVE ON

3 THINGS I AM THANKFUL FOR LAST 24 HOURS:

1. _____

2. _____

3. _____

THOUGHT DOWNLOAD

NOTES

AFFIRMATION OF THE DAY: --

TODAY, I AM LOOKING FORWARD TO

GOALS #1	GOALS #2	HABITS I AM TRACKING	Y/N

THOUGHT DOWNLOAD

TODAY I AM CHOOSING TO FEEL:

C -

T -

F -
A -

R -

I WILL DRINK ___ GLASSES OF WATER TODAY: 1 2 3 4 5 6 7 8 9 10

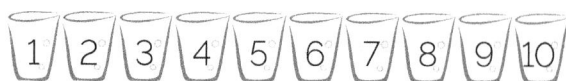

JENNIFER BULBROOK

LOOKING BACK ON MY AMAZINGNESS

MY WINS I CELEBRATE TODAY ARE	TOMORROW I WILL IMPROVE ON

3 THINGS I AM THANKFUL FOR LAST 24 HOURS:

1. ______________________________

2. ______________________________

3. ______________________________

THOUGHT DOWNLOAD

NOTES

AFFIRMATION OF THE DAY: _____

TODAY, I AM LOOKING FORWARD TO

GOALS #1	GOALS #2

HABITS I AM TRACKING	Y/N

THOUGHT DOWNLOAD

TODAY I AM CHOOSING TO FEEL:

C -

T -

F -
A -

R -

I WILL DRINK ___ GLASSES OF WATER TODAY: 1 2 3 4 5 6 7 8 9 10

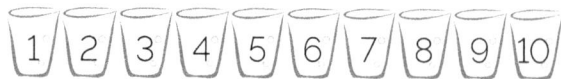

LOOKING BACK ON MY AMAZINGNESS

MY WINS I CELEBRATE TODAY ARE	TOMORROW I WILL IMPROVE ON

3 THINGS I AM THANKFUL FOR LAST 24 HOURS:

1. ____________________

2. ____________________

3. ____________________

THOUGHT DOWNLOAD

NOTES

AFFIRMATION OF THE DAY: _____

TODAY, I AM LOOKING FORWARD TO

GOALS #1	GOALS #2	HABITS I AM TRACKING	Y/N

THOUGHT DOWNLOAD

TODAY I AM CHOOSING TO FEEL:

C -

T -

F -
A -

R -

I WILL DRINK ___ GLASSES OF WATER TODAY: 1 2 3 4 5 6 7 8 9 10

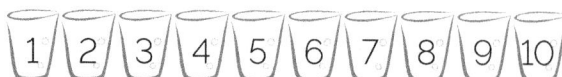

LOOKING BACK ON MY AMAZINGNESS

MY WINS I CELEBRATE TODAY ARE	TOMORROW I WILL IMPROVE ON

3 THINGS I AM THANKFUL FOR LAST 24 HOURS:

1. ______________________________

2. ______________________________

3. ______________________________

THOUGHT DOWNLOAD

NOTES

AFFIRMATION OF THE DAY: _____

TODAY, I AM LOOKING FORWARD TO

GOALS #1

GOALS #2

HABITS I AM TRACKING	Y/N

THOUGHT DOWNLOAD

TODAY I AM CHOOSING TO FEEL:

C -

T -

F -
A -

R -

I WILL DRINK ___ GLASSES OF WATER TODAY: 1 2 3 4 5 6 7 8 9 10

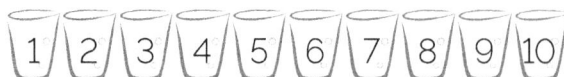

LOOKING BACK ON MY AMAZINGNESS

MY WINS I CELEBRATE TODAY ARE	TOMORROW I WILL IMPROVE ON

3 THINGS I AM THANKFUL FOR LAST 24 HOURS:

1. ____________________

2. ____________________

3. ____________________

THOUGHT DOWNLOAD

NOTES

AFFIRMATION OF THE DAY: _____

TODAY, I AM LOOKING FORWARD TO

GOALS #1	GOALS #2	HABITS I AM TRACKING	Y/N

THOUGHT DOWNLOAD

TODAY I AM CHOOSING TO FEEL:

C -

T -

F -
A -

R -

I WILL DRINK ___ GLASSES OF WATER TODAY: 1 2 3 4 5 6 7 8 9 10

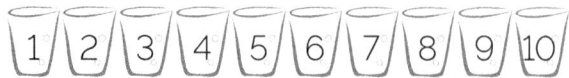

MY WINS I CELEBRATE TODAY ARE	TOMORROW I WILL IMPROVE ON

3 THINGS I AM THANKFUL FOR LAST 24 HOURS:

1. _____

2. _____

3. _____

THOUGHT DOWNLOAD

NOTES

MY WEEK OF AWESOMENESS!
Now that our yearly and monthly goals are done, we now can break down
our goals even further to make them even more achievable

REFLECTIONS OF LAST WEEK:

OBSTACLES I MAY FACE: _____

_____

SOLUTIONS: _____

_____

MY WEEK OF_____

Task- write "I Am Amazing because and then list all the amazing things about you.

TIME	MONDAY [ ]	TUESDAY [ ]	WEDNESDAY [ ]

MY WEEK OF AWESOMENESS!

6 Month Goal	6 Month Goal
MONTH	MONTH
WEEK	WEEK
REWARD WHEN I REACH	REWARD WHEN I REACH

MY WEEK OF _____

What time do you want to wake up at, go to bed? How do you want your week to look like?
What events or meetings do you need to attend? Are you planning on having a day of shopping?

THURSDAY [ ]	FRIDAY [ ]	SATURDAY [ ]	SUNDAY [ ]

THERE IS NOT PERFECTION!

AFFIRMATION OF THE DAY: _____

TODAY, I AM LOOKING FORWARD TO

GOALS #1	GOALS #2

HABITS I AM TRACKING	Y/N

THOUGHT DOWNLOAD

TODAY I AM CHOOSING TO FEEL:

C -

T -

F -
A -

R -

I WILL DRINK ___ GLASSES OF WATER TODAY: 1 2 3 4 5 6 7 8 9 10

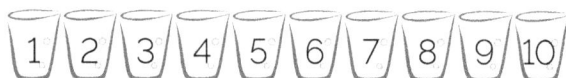

LOOKING BACK ON MY AMAZINGNESS

MY WINS I CELEBRATE TODAY ARE	TOMORROW I WILL IMPROVE ON

3 THINGS I AM THANKFUL FOR LAST 24 HOURS:

1. ______

2. ______

3. ______

THOUGHT DOWNLOAD

NOTES

AFFIRMATION OF THE DAY: _____

TODAY, I AM LOOKING FORWARD TO

GOALS #1	GOALS #2	HABITS I AM TRACKING	Y/N

THOUGHT DOWNLOAD

TODAY I AM CHOOSING TO FEEL:

C -

T -

F -
A -

R -

I WILL DRINK ___ GLASSES OF WATER TODAY: 1 2 3 4 5 6 7 8 9 10

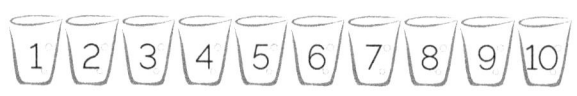

LOOKING BACK ON MY AMAZINGNESS

MY WINS I CELEBRATE TODAY ARE	TOMORROW I WILL IMPROVE ON

3 THINGS I AM THANKFUL FOR LAST 24 HOURS:

1. ______________________________

2. ______________________________

3. ______________________________

THOUGHT DOWNLOAD

NOTES

AFFIRMATION OF THE DAY: _____

TODAY, I AM LOOKING FORWARD TO

GOALS #1	GOALS #2	HABITS I AM TRACKING	Y/N

THOUGHT DOWNLOAD

TODAY I AM CHOOSING TO FEEL:

C -

T -

F -
A -

R -

I WILL DRINK ___ GLASSES OF WATER TODAY: 1 2 3 4 5 6 7 8 9 10

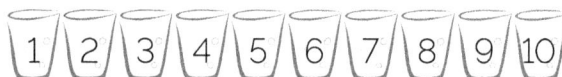

LOOKING BACK ON MY AMAZINGNESS

MY WINS I CELEBRATE TODAY ARE	TOMORROW I WILL IMPROVE ON

3 THINGS I AM THANKFUL FOR LAST 24 HOURS:

1. ______________________________

2. ______________________________

3. ______________________________

THOUGHT DOWNLOAD

NOTES

AFFIRMATION OF THE DAY: _____

TODAY, I AM LOOKING FORWARD TO

GOALS #1	GOALS #2	HABITS I AM TRACKING	Y/N

THOUGHT DOWNLOAD

TODAY I AM CHOOSING TO FEEL:

C -

T -

F -
A -

R -

I WILL DRINK ___ GLASSES OF WATER TODAY: 1 2 3 4 5 6 7 8 9 10

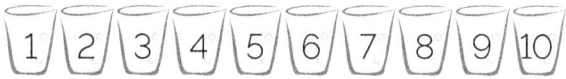

LOOKING BACK ON MY AMAZINGNESS

MY WINS I CELEBRATE TODAY ARE	TOMORROW I WILL IMPROVE ON

3 THINGS I AM THANKFUL FOR LAST 24 HOURS:

1. _____

2. _____

3. _____

THOUGHT DOWNLOAD

NOTES

AFFIRMATION OF THE DAY: _____

TODAY, I AM LOOKING FORWARD TO

GOALS #1	GOALS #2	HABITS I AM TRACKING	Y/N

THOUGHT DOWNLOAD

TODAY I AM CHOOSING TO FEEL:

C -

T -

F -
A -

R -

I WILL DRINK ___ GLASSES OF WATER TODAY: 1 2 3 4 5 6 7 8 9 10

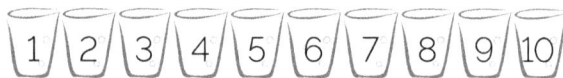

LOOKING BACK ON MY AMAZINGNESS

MY WINS I CELEBRATE TODAY ARE	TOMORROW I WILL IMPROVE ON

3 THINGS I AM THANKFUL FOR LAST 24 HOURS:

1. _____

2. _____

3. _____

THOUGHT DOWNLOAD

NOTES

AFFIRMATION OF THE DAY: _____

TODAY, I AM LOOKING FORWARD TO

GOALS #1	GOALS #2

HABITS I AM TRACKING	Y/N

THOUGHT DOWNLOAD

TODAY I AM CHOOSING TO FEEL:

C -

T -

F -
A -

R -

I WILL DRINK ___ GLASSES OF WATER TODAY: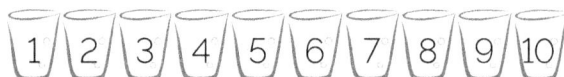

LOOKING BACK ON MY AMAZINGNESS

MY WINS I CELEBRATE TODAY ARE	TOMORROW I WILL IMPROVE ON

3 THINGS I AM THANKFUL FOR LAST 24 HOURS:

1. ______________________________

2. ______________________________

3. ______________________________

THOUGHT DOWNLOAD

NOTES

AFFIRMATION OF THE DAY: ---

TODAY, I AM LOOKING FORWARD TO

GOALS #1	GOALS #2

HABITS I AM TRACKING	Y/N

THOUGHT DOWNLOAD

TODAY I AM CHOOSING TO FEEL:

C -

T -

F -
A -

R -

I WILL DRINK ___ GLASSES OF WATER TODAY: 1 2 3 4 5 6 7 8 9 10

LOOKING BACK ON MY AMAZINGNESS

MY WINS I CELEBRATE TODAY ARE	TOMORROW I WILL IMPROVE ON

3 THINGS I AM THANKFUL FOR LAST 24 HOURS:

1. ______________________________

2. ______________________________

3. ______________________________

THOUGHT DOWNLOAD

NOTES

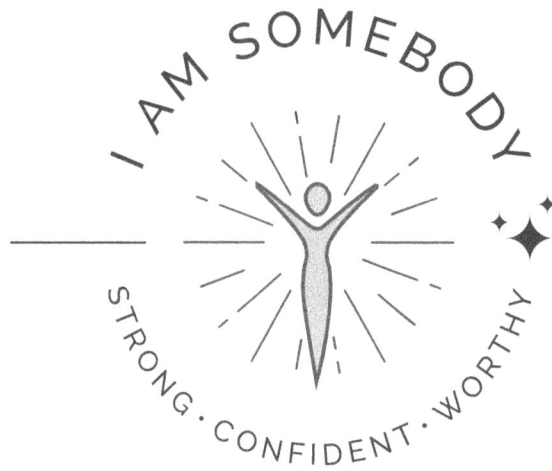

I AM SOMBODY

Transform Your Life Organizer™

Month Five

SELF-ESTEEM

When I first started my research for this **Transform Your Life Organizer ™**, I thought, ok this will be easy, I know what self-worth means. I can explain this easily. Well, I was wrong, and as I read about self-worth I realized it is a little more complex, and it's not the same thing as self esteem or self confidence. These are all subjects on their own and I will be speaking about throughout your journey. Our main goal with this organizer is to make sure you walk away knowing you are worthy, and You Are Somebody.

Self-esteem and self-confidence are tied into our self-worth and to have a high sense of self-worth we must accept ourselves completely, the good, "the flaws", everything and that is what we will be working on over the next few weeks.

To build our self-worth, we must build our self-esteem, be aware and accept who we are. Our self-esteem is what we think, feel, and believe about ourselves and are lucky for us, we are the ones in control of our own self esteem. How cool is that?

How we think about ourselves begins at a young age, we can not blame how we think or feel on what we were taught or went through growing up. Whether we have had a shitty childhood or told some negative things as a child, or by our own children, we get to decide how we think and feel about ourselves.

To increase our self esteem, there are several things we can do:

1. Think positive

2. Positive affirmations

3. Do not compare yourself to others

4. Live in the present

5. Keep on track daily of your personal hygiene, including clean clothes

6. Learn to accept compliments

7. Have self-care days where you do something for yourself like a spa day or fishing with the boys

8. Make lists of your strengths, the things you love about yourself, your achievements, what compliments you get from others

9. Take care of yourself physically

Please note, you need to do these things repeatedly, not a "done once and fixed". It does not work like magic, there is no quick fix, but it will take time, commitment, and hard work. You CAN and WILL do it.

You must believe that you have high self-esteem to feel the feelings and go through this exercise to produce a result. Now if you do not believe it yet and it's just to far out of reach still, that's ok. Just modify your thoughts to something that you CAN believe, like "I have self-esteem", or "my self esteem has grown so much."

TASK: Now, I want you to imagine having extremely high self-esteem or like I mentioned, modify that thought if needed. How do you feel? What can you see? How can you feel physically? What do you think? How has your life changed?

Practice loving yourself, practice loving the parts that you do not like about yourself.

List 100 things you appreciate about yourself

Thinking something wrong with ourselves is a choice.

SELF-CONFIDENCE

Google's definition is a feeling of trust in one's own abilities, qualities, and judgments. Self- confidence shows in everything we do and who would not want self-confidence, but the truth is, not everyone is willing to create it. I have often heard people (including me) say things like:

"I wish I were confident like them."

"I wish I felt comfortable enough to just be me."

"I wish I did not feel like I needed a drink to be sociable."

"I wish I could make a room turn; like they do."

"I wish I was confident enough to begin my own business and to show the world my ideas, etc."

People say these things all the time however very rarely do they do anything to change or gain the confidence that they have been longing for.

The subconscious mind works with the information we give it by translating our thoughts into reality whether based on fear or courage and therefore it does not differentiate between what is real and what is imagined. The good news is… because the way we see ourselves is simply a figure that we made up of with a collection of our thoughts, we can therefore change those thoughts which ultimately will change our self-confidence. For many years I told myself I was not good enough; that I could never share my ideas with anyone and what do I know anyway? Who is going to listen to me? The list of self-doubt, negative self-talk and discouraging myself for years destroyed any self-confidence I did have. Once I began my journey of self-worth, I began to build my self-confidence. Now when I look at myself, I see that I've built my own Brand; and that I am sharing so many of my ideas with the world. I am accomplishing amazing things and feeling wonderful about myself. I can now say and believe that I am good enough. I DO know what I am talking about. People not only want to listen to me, but they do. I am great. I am beautiful. I love me.

It takes a real commitment and a strong desire. You cannot expect to build confidence just by sitting around thinking good thoughts. You must believe in your ability to get what you want no matter what you need to learn or how many times you try or fail. Self-confidence fuels action so believe you can do it, believe that it will work out, believe that you have the capability, believe you are worth it, believe you Are Somebody and act. As soon as you do, the fear on the inside will begin to decrease and your confidence will increase. Sure, there will be mistakes along the way, that is to be expected, it is not the end of the world. In fact, it is when our mindset grows the most.

We should not allow our self-confidence to be determined by outside factors. If we base our self-confidence on how well we play pool and then someone else comes along and plays better, does that mean my self-confidence should decrease? Hell, no, but if you are determining your self- confidence from those outside factors then, then that is what will happen. In other words, if you want to gain self-confidence, start by feeding your mind with tons of thoughts of self-love that come from within. Self-confidence comes with feeling, experiencing all your emotions.

SELF-WORTH

How much time do you take each day choosing you? Do you find that after a long day of making time for everyone else and with work you are just exhausted and end up spending the remainder of your time distracting yourself with social media or binge-watching some show? Well, today that stops as you DESERVE much more than that, so no matter what you have going on in your life, today you are going to begin prioritizing YOU because you are worth it. Say it with me… **"I AM SOMEBODY"!**

The most important decision you will make in your life is deciding that you want to believe in your worthiness. Make your worthiness non-negotiable. The second most important decision is to pass along that belief to the other people in your life because we are all worthy and deserve the same amount of attention, love, and respect as one another.

I have recently begun to think and believe that I am amazing, and it really has helped me so much to elevate my self-esteem and worth. Not only do I know you are amazing, but I believe you are amazing too. You are probably thinking "how can she say that she does not even know me?"

I know this because we all are born worthy and no matter what we say or do, that does not change. There is nothing I can do or say that will make me less worthy and the same goes for everyone. Some of us may forget we are worthy because of a vicious pattern of negative thoughts about ourselves that are getting in the way.

How we think about things and what we believe is what ultimately controls our actions and has a huge impact on our self-confidence. Believing you are not good enough limits you from reaching your fullest potential. Becoming aware and examining your thoughts is key.

What's holding you back?

Is it your false belief that you are nobody? Is it your false belief that you do not deserve what you want? Is it your false belief that you are not worthy? If this is the case, it is time to question, dispose and replace those limiting beliefs with the truth that you are worthy of achieving your goals and that You Are Somebody!

When we are have negative beliefs, whether it is about how we look, our abilities, how we do something, our lives, past, no matter what it is, we need to replace those beliefs with ones that are true and will serve us. We all have a choice as to what we believe about life and about ourselves. I choose to believe in myself, I choose to believe in the process and know that I am evolving each day that I show up. What do you choose to believe?

WHAT DOES NOT DETERMINE SELF-WORTH:

- **People:** You and your personal achievements are more important than what others are thinking, saying, or doing. Do NOT compare yourself with other people; just focus on being you, the best you. Just like there cannot be another one of you, there cannot be another one of him or her so stop trying to be like anyone but yourself.

- **Friends:** The number of friends or people you know has absolutely nothing to do with your worth as a human.

- **Relationship status:** Your self-worth does not shift based on whether you are single, married, divorced, or widowed.

- **Social Media:** It does not matter how many followers or likes you receive or how many people comment, your worth is not measured by social media.

- **Job/Career:** All that matters is that you work, you work hard, you do so to the best to your abilities and most importantly, that you enjoy doing.

- **Money:** Sure, money is great, who does not love money? But money does not define you. No matter how much money you have (or don't have), you are still you.

- **Likes/Tastes/Enjoyments:** It doesn't matter if you shop at the finest shops or at second-hand stores. Your worth is the same either way. It does not matter if you enjoy sports or if you prefer the Opera. Your worth does not change.

- **To-Do-List:** Your goals don't define you either, you are not your goals. Yes, achieving your goals feels amazing, but it does not define who you are.

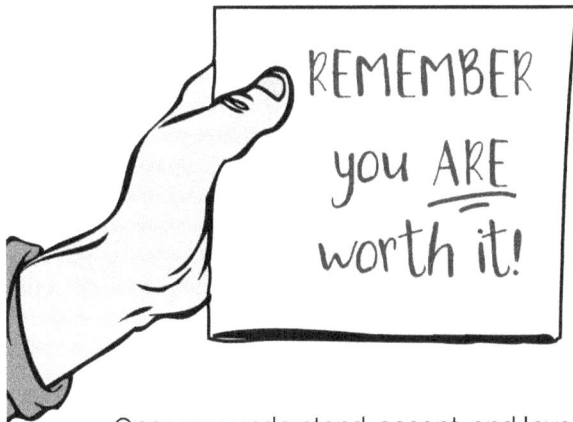

REMEMBER you ARE worth it!

WE ALL ARE WORTH IT EQUALLY. WE ARE BORN WORTHY! RECOGNIZING YOUR SELF-WORTH

Once you understand, accept, and love yourself, you will reach a point where you no longer depend on external factors like people and accomplishments for your self-worth.

At this point, the best thing you can do is recognize your worth and appreciate yourself for the work you have done to get here, as well as continuing to maintain your self-understanding, self-acceptance, self-love, and self-worth.

To recognize your self-worth, remind yourself that:

1. You no longer need to please others.

2.. No matter what others do or say, you alone have control over how you feel about yourself.

3.. Regardless of what happens outside of you, you are in control of yourself and how you feel and do things.

4.. You have the power to control how you respond to all outside factors.

5.. Your worth comes from inside, we are all born worthy, and we never lose that worth, we just sometimes think differently.

1. Things I am good at:

2. What I like about my appearance:

3. I have helped others by:

4. Challenges I have overcome:

5. Things that make me unique:

6. Times I have made others happy:

7. My personality is:

Your belief in your Self-Worth will factor in successes and failures in life.
If you want to improve on anything in your life it is important to explore
what is going on inside and to evaluate what you're thinking.

MONTHLY GOALS

WOO-HOO YOU FINISHED ANOTHER MONTH:

"You yourself, as much as anybody in the entire universe, deserve your love and affection." Buddha

6 MONTHS GOAL	MONTHLY GOAL
GOAL #1	
GOAL #2	

MONTH AT A GLANCE -

FACE AND WALK THROUGH ONE OF YOUR FEARS

NOTES			

THEN, FACE ANOTHER AND ANOTHER. YOUR SELF- ESTEEM WILL INCREASE!

Every Sunday review & re-evaluate your goals. Identify obstacles that you faced, along with solutions.

		TAKE PRIDE IN YOUR APPEARANCE ALL THE TIME NO MATTER WHERE YOU ARE!	Say it with me… I AM SOMEBODY

MY WEEK OF AWESOMENESS!
Now that 6 month and monthly goals are done, we now can break down
our goals even further to make them even more achievable

REFLECTIONS OF LAST WEEK:

OBSTACLES I MAY FACE: _____

_____

SOLUTIONS: _____

_____

MY WEEK OF_____
Take 1-5 days this month to go through all your belongings and what you do not use regularly or have multiple of them is time to part with them. When parting with anything that is not actual trash, donate or sell these items.

TIME			

MY WEEK OF AWESOMENESS!

6 Month Goal	6 Month Goal
MONTH	MONTH
WEEK	WEEK
REWARD WHEN I REACH	REWARD WHEN I REACH

MY WEEK OF _____

What time do you want to wake up at, go to bed? How do you want your week to look like?

What events or meetings do you need to attend? Are you planning on having a day of shopping?

AFFIRMATION OF THE DAY: _____

TODAY, I AM LOOKING FORWARD TO

GOALS #1	GOALS #2	HABITS I AM TRACKING	Y/N

THOUGHT DOWNLOAD

TODAY I AM CHOOSING TO FEEL:

C -

T -

F -
A -

R -

I WILL DRINK ___ GLASSES OF WATER TODAY: 1 2 3 4 5 6 7 8 9 10

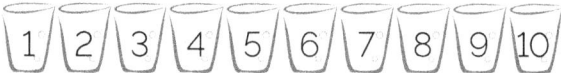

LOOKING BACK ON MY AMAZINGNESS

MY WINS I CELEBRATE TODAY ARE	TOMORROW I WILL IMPROVE ON

3 THINGS I AM THANKFUL FOR LAST 24 HOURS:

1. ______________________________

2. ______________________________

3. ______________________________

THOUGHT DOWNLOAD

NOTES

AFFIRMATION OF THE DAY: _____

TODAY, I AM LOOKING FORWARD TO

GOALS #1	GOALS #2

HABITS I AM TRACKING	Y/N

THOUGHT DOWNLOAD

TODAY I AM CHOOSING TO FEEL:

C -

T -

F -
A -

R -

I WILL DRINK ___ GLASSES OF WATER TODAY: 1 2 3 4 5 6 7 8 9 10

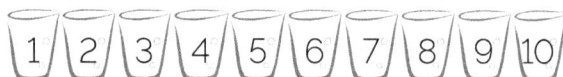

LOOKING BACK ON MY AMAZINGNESS

MY WINS I CELEBRATE TODAY ARE	TOMORROW I WILL IMPROVE ON

3 THINGS I AM THANKFUL FOR LAST 24 HOURS:

1. ______________________________

2. ______________________________

3. ______________________________

THOUGHT DOWNLOAD

NOTES

AFFIRMATION OF THE DAY: --

TODAY, I AM LOOKING FORWARD TO

GOALS #1	GOALS #2	HABITS I AM TRACKING	Y/N

THOUGHT DOWNLOAD

TODAY I AM CHOOSING TO FEEL:

C -

T -

F -
A -

R -

I WILL DRINK ___ GLASSES OF WATER TODAY: 1 2 3 4 5 6 7 8 9 10

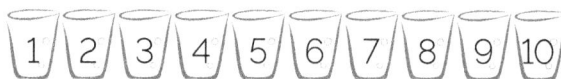

LOOKING BACK ON MY AMAZINGNESS

MY WINS I CELEBRATE TODAY ARE	TOMORROW I WILL IMPROVE ON

3 THINGS I AM THANKFUL FOR LAST 24 HOURS:

1. ______________________________

2. ______________________________

3. ______________________________

THOUGHT DOWNLOAD

NOTES

AFFIRMATION OF THE DAY: _____

TODAY, I AM LOOKING FORWARD TO

GOALS #1	GOALS #2	HABITS I AM TRACKING	Y/N

THOUGHT DOWNLOAD

TODAY I AM CHOOSING TO FEEL:

C -

T -

F -
A -

R -

I WILL DRINK ___ GLASSES OF WATER TODAY: 1 2 3 4 5 6 7 8 9 10

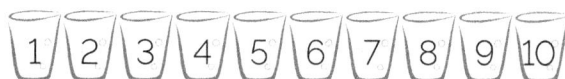

LOOKING BACK ON MY AMAZINGNESS

MY WINS I CELEBRATE TODAY ARE	TOMORROW I WILL IMPROVE ON

3 THINGS I AM THANKFUL FOR LAST 24 HOURS:

1. ______________________________

2. ______________________________

3. ______________________________

THOUGHT DOWNLOAD

NOTES

AFFIRMATION OF THE DAY: --

TODAY, I AM LOOKING FORWARD TO

GOALS #1	GOALS #2	HABITS I AM TRACKING	Y/N

THOUGHT DOWNLOAD

TODAY I AM CHOOSING TO FEEL:

C -

T -

F -
A -

R -

I WILL DRINK ___ GLASSES OF WATER TODAY: 1 2 3 4 5 6 7 8 9 10

LOOKING BACK ON MY AMAZINGNESS

MY WINS I CELEBRATE TODAY ARE	TOMORROW I WILL IMPROVE ON

3 THINGS I AM THANKFUL FOR LAST 24 HOURS:

1. ____________________

2. ____________________

3. ____________________

THOUGHT DOWNLOAD

NOTES

AFFIRMATION OF THE DAY: _____

TODAY, I AM LOOKING FORWARD TO

GOALS #1	GOALS #2	HABITS I AM TRACKING	Y/N

THOUGHT DOWNLOAD

TODAY I AM CHOOSING TO FEEL:

C -

T -

F -
A -

R -

I WILL DRINK ___ GLASSES OF WATER TODAY: 1 2 3 4 5 6 7 8 9 10

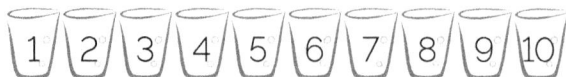

LOOKING BACK ON MY AMAZINGNESS

MY WINS I CELEBRATE TODAY ARE	TOMORROW I WILL IMPROVE ON

3 THINGS I AM THANKFUL FOR LAST 24 HOURS:

1. ______________________________

2. ______________________________

3. ______________________________

THOUGHT DOWNLOAD

NOTES

AFFIRMATION OF THE DAY: _____

TODAY, I AM LOOKING FORWARD TO

GOALS #1	GOALS #2

HABITS I AM TRACKING	Y/N

THOUGHT DOWNLOAD

TODAY I AM CHOOSING TO FEEL:

C -

T -

F -
A -

R -

I WILL DRINK ___ GLASSES OF WATER TODAY: 1 2 3 4 5 6 7 8 9 10

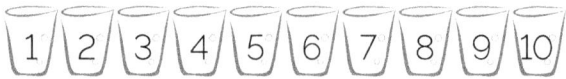

MY WINS I CELEBRATE TODAY ARE	TOMORROW I WILL IMPROVE ON

3 THINGS I AM THANKFUL FOR LAST 24 HOURS:

1. _____

2. _____

3. _____

THOUGHT DOWNLOAD

NOTES

MY WEEK OF AWESOMENESS!
Now that 6 month and monthly goals are done, we now can break down
our goals even further to make them even more achievable

REFLECTIONS OF LAST WEEK:

OBSTACLES I MAY FACE: _____

_____

SOLUTIONS: _____

_____

MY WEEK OF_____
Take 1-5 days this month to go through all your belongings and what you do not use regularly or have multiple of
them is time to part with them. When parting with anything that is not actual trash, donate or sell these items.

TIME			

MY WEEK OF AWESOMENESS!

6 Month Goal	6 Month Goal
MONTH	MONTH
WEEK	WEEK
REWARD WHEN I REACH	REWARD WHEN I REACH

MY WEEK OF_____

What time do you want to wake up at, go to bed? How do you want your week to look like?
What events or meetings do you need to attend? Are you planning on having a day of shopping?

AFFIRMATION OF THE DAY: _____

TODAY, I AM LOOKING FORWARD TO

GOALS #1	GOALS #2	HABITS I AM TRACKING	Y/N

THOUGHT DOWNLOAD

TODAY I AM CHOOSING TO FEEL:

C -

T -

F -
A -

R -

 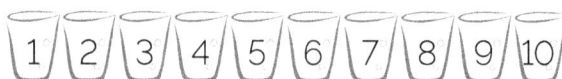

JENNIFER BULBROOK

LOOKING BACK ON MY AMAZINGNESS

MY WINS I CELEBRATE TODAY ARE	TOMORROW I WILL IMPROVE ON

3 THINGS I AM THANKFUL FOR LAST 24 HOURS:

1. ______________________________

2. ______________________________

3. ______________________________

THOUGHT DOWNLOAD

NOTES

AFFIRMATION OF THE DAY: _____

TODAY, I AM LOOKING FORWARD TO

GOALS #1	GOALS #2	HABITS I AM TRACKING	Y/N

THOUGHT DOWNLOAD

TODAY I AM CHOOSING TO FEEL:

C -

T -

F -
A -

R -

I WILL DRINK ___ GLASSES OF WATER TODAY: 1 2 3 4 5 6 7 8 9 10

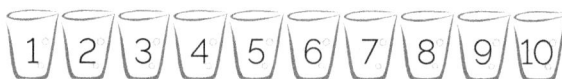

LOOKING BACK ON MY AMAZINGNESS

MY WINS I CELEBRATE TODAY ARE	TOMORROW I WILL IMPROVE ON

3 THINGS I AM THANKFUL FOR LAST 24 HOURS:

1. ______________________________

2. ______________________________

3. ______________________________

THOUGHT DOWNLOAD

NOTES

AFFIRMATION OF THE DAY: _____

TODAY, I AM LOOKING FORWARD TO

GOALS #1	GOALS #2	HABITS I AM TRACKING	Y/N

THOUGHT DOWNLOAD

TODAY I AM CHOOSING TO FEEL:

C -

T -

F -
A -

R -

I WILL DRINK ___ GLASSES OF WATER TODAY: 1 2 3 4 5 6 7 8 9 10

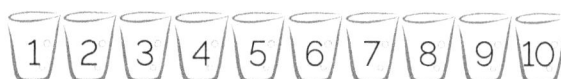

LOOKING BACK ON MY AMAZINGNESS

MY WINS I CELEBRATE TODAY ARE   TOMORROW I WILL IMPROVE ON

3 THINGS I AM THANKFUL FOR LAST 24 HOURS:

1. _____

2. _____

3. _____

THOUGHT DOWNLOAD

NOTES

AFFIRMATION OF THE DAY: _____

TODAY, I AM LOOKING FORWARD TO

GOALS #1	GOALS #2	HABITS I AM TRACKING	Y/N

THOUGHT DOWNLOAD

TODAY I AM CHOOSING TO FEEL:

C -

T -

F -
A -

R -

I WILL DRINK ___ GLASSES OF WATER TODAY: 1 2 3 4 5 6 7 8 9 10

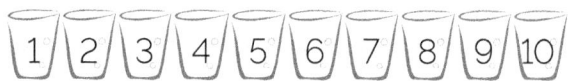

LOOKING BACK ON MY AMAZINGNESS

MY WINS I CELEBRATE TODAY ARE	TOMORROW I WILL IMPROVE ON

3 THINGS I AM THANKFUL FOR LAST 24 HOURS:

1. _____

2. _____

3. _____

THOUGHT DOWNLOAD

NOTES

AFFIRMATION OF THE DAY: _____

TODAY, I AM LOOKING FORWARD TO

GOALS #1	GOALS #2

HABITS I AM TRACKING	Y/N

THOUGHT DOWNLOAD

TODAY I AM CHOOSING TO FEEL:

C -

T -

F -
A -

R -

I WILL DRINK ___ GLASSES OF WATER TODAY: 1 2 3 4 5 6 7 8 9 10

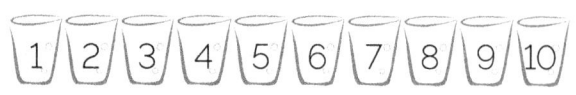

JENNIFER BULBROOK

LOOKING BACK ON MY AMAZINGNESS

MY WINS I CELEBRATE TODAY ARE	TOMORROW I WILL IMPROVE ON

3 THINGS I AM THANKFUL FOR LAST 24 HOURS:

1. ______________________________

2. ______________________________

3. ______________________________

THOUGHT DOWNLOAD

NOTES

AFFIRMATION OF THE DAY: _____

TODAY, I AM LOOKING FORWARD TO

GOALS #1	GOALS #2	HABITS I AM TRACKING	Y/N

THOUGHT DOWNLOAD

TODAY I AM CHOOSING TO FEEL:

C -

T -

F -
A -

R -

I WILL DRINK ___ GLASSES OF WATER TODAY: 1 2 3 4 5 6 7 8 9 10

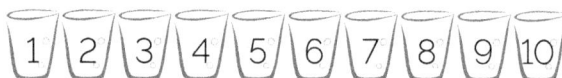

LOOKING BACK ON MY AMAZINGNESS

MY WINS I CELEBRATE TODAY ARE	TOMORROW I WILL IMPROVE ON

3 THINGS I AM THANKFUL FOR LAST 24 HOURS:

1. ______________________________

2. ______________________________

3. ______________________________

THOUGHT DOWNLOAD

NOTES

AFFIRMATION OF THE DAY: _____

TODAY, I AM LOOKING FORWARD TO

GOALS #1	GOALS #2	HABITS I AM TRACKING	Y/N

THOUGHT DOWNLOAD

TODAY I AM CHOOSING TO FEEL:

C -

T -

F -
A -

R -

I WILL DRINK ___ GLASSES OF WATER TODAY: 1 2 3 4 5 6 7 8 9 10

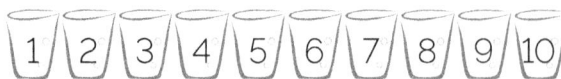

LOOKING BACK ON MY AMAZINGNESS

MY WINS I CELEBRATE TODAY ARE	TOMORROW I WILL IMPROVE ON

3 THINGS I AM THANKFUL FOR LAST 24 HOURS:

1. _____

2. _____

3. _____

THOUGHT DOWNLOAD

NOTES

MY WEEK OF AWESOMENESS!
Now that 6 month and monthly goals are done, we now can break down our goals even further to make them even more achievable

REFLECTIONS OF LAST WEEK:

OBSTACLES I MAY FACE: _____

_____

SOLUTIONS: _____

_____

MY WEEK OF_____
Take 1-5 days this month to go through all your belongings and what you do not use regularly or have multiple of them is time to part with them. When parting with anything that is not actual trash, donate or sell these items.

TIME			

JENNIFER BULBROOK

MY WEEK OF AWESOMENESS!

6 Month Goal	6 Month Goal
MONTH	MONTH
WEEK	WEEK
REWARD WHEN I REACH	REWARD WHEN I REACH

MY WEEK OF_____

What time do you want to wake up at, go to bed? How do you want your week to look like?
What events or meetings do you need to attend? Are you planning on having a day of shopping?

AFFIRMATION OF THE DAY: ---

TODAY, I AM LOOKING FORWARD TO

GOALS #1	GOALS #2	HABITS I AM TRACKING	Y/N

THOUGHT DOWNLOAD

TODAY I AM CHOOSING TO FEEL:

C -

T -

F -
A -

R -

I WILL DRINK ___ GLASSES OF WATER TODAY: 1 2 3 4 5 6 7 8 9 10

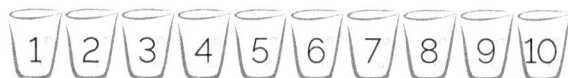

LOOKING BACK ON MY AMAZINGNESS

MY WINS I CELEBRATE TODAY ARE	TOMORROW I WILL IMPROVE ON

3 THINGS I AM THANKFUL FOR LAST 24 HOURS:

1. ______________________________

2. ______________________________

3. ______________________________

THOUGHT DOWNLOAD

NOTES

AFFIRMATION OF THE DAY: _____

TODAY, I AM LOOKING FORWARD TO

GOALS #1

GOALS #2

HABITS I AM TRACKING	Y/N

THOUGHT DOWNLOAD

TODAY I AM CHOOSING TO FEEL:

C -

T -

F -
A -

R -

I WILL DRINK ___ GLASSES OF WATER TODAY: 1 2 3 4 5 6 7 8 9 10

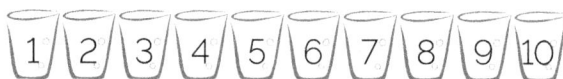

LOOKING BACK ON MY AMAZINGNESS

MY WINS I CELEBRATE TODAY ARE	TOMORROW I WILL IMPROVE ON

3 THINGS I AM THANKFUL FOR LAST 24 HOURS:

1. ______________________________

2. ______________________________

3. ______________________________

THOUGHT DOWNLOAD

NOTES

AFFIRMATION OF THE DAY: _____

TODAY, I AM LOOKING FORWARD TO

GOALS #1	GOALS #2

HABITS I AM TRACKING	Y/N

THOUGHT DOWNLOAD

TODAY I AM CHOOSING TO FEEL:

C -

T -

F -
A -

R -

I WILL DRINK ___ GLASSES OF WATER TODAY: 1 2 3 4 5 6 7 8 9 10

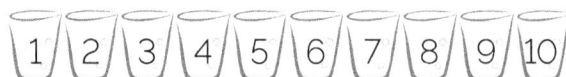

LOOKING BACK ON MY AMAZINGNESS

MY WINS I CELEBRATE TODAY ARE	TOMORROW I WILL IMPROVE ON

3 THINGS I AM THANKFUL FOR LAST 24 HOURS:

1. ______________________________

2. ______________________________

3. ______________________________

THOUGHT DOWNLOAD

NOTES

AFFIRMATION OF THE DAY: _____

TODAY, I AM LOOKING FORWARD TO

GOALS #1	GOALS #2

HABITS I AM TRACKING	Y/N

THOUGHT DOWNLOAD

TODAY I AM CHOOSING TO FEEL:

C -

T -

F -
A -

R -

I WILL DRINK ___ GLASSES OF WATER TODAY: 1 2 3 4 5 6 7 8 9 10

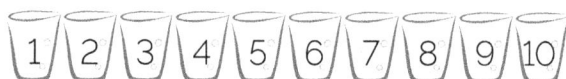

LOOKING BACK ON MY AMAZINGNESS

MY WINS I CELEBRATE TODAY ARE	TOMORROW I WILL IMPROVE ON

3 THINGS I AM THANKFUL FOR LAST 24 HOURS:

1. ______________________________

2. ______________________________

3. ______________________________

THOUGHT DOWNLOAD

NOTES

AFFIRMATION OF THE DAY: _____

TODAY, I AM LOOKING FORWARD TO

GOALS #1

GOALS #2

HABITS I AM TRACKING	Y/N

THOUGHT DOWNLOAD

TODAY I AM CHOOSING TO FEEL:

C -

T -

F -
A -

R -

I WILL DRINK ___ GLASSES OF WATER TODAY: 1 2 3 4 5 6 7 8 9 10

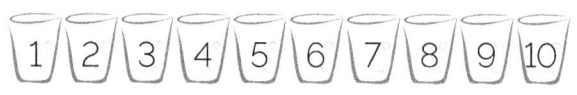

LOOKING BACK ON MY AMAZINGNESS

MY WINS I CELEBRATE TODAY ARE	TOMORROW I WILL IMPROVE ON

3 THINGS I AM THANKFUL FOR LAST 24 HOURS:

1. ______________________________

2. ______________________________

3. ______________________________

THOUGHT DOWNLOAD

NOTES

AFFIRMATION OF THE DAY: _____

TODAY, I AM LOOKING FORWARD TO

GOALS #1	GOALS #2	HABITS I AM TRACKING	Y/N

THOUGHT DOWNLOAD

TODAY I AM CHOOSING TO FEEL:

C -

T -

F -
A -

R -

I WILL DRINK ___ GLASSES OF WATER TODAY: 1 2 3 4 5 6 7 8 9 10

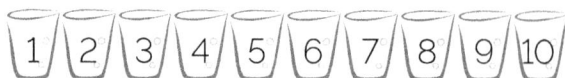

LOOKING BACK ON MY AMAZINGNESS

MY WINS I CELEBRATE TODAY ARE	TOMORROW I WILL IMPROVE ON

3 THINGS I AM THANKFUL FOR LAST 24 HOURS:

1. ____________________

2. ____________________

3. ____________________

THOUGHT DOWNLOAD

NOTES

AFFIRMATION OF THE DAY: _____

TODAY, I AM LOOKING FORWARD TO

GOALS #1	GOALS #2

HABITS I AM TRACKING	Y/N

THOUGHT DOWNLOAD

TODAY I AM CHOOSING TO FEEL:

C -

T -

F -
A -

R -

I WILL DRINK ___ GLASSES OF WATER TODAY: 1 2 3 4 5 6 7 8 9 10

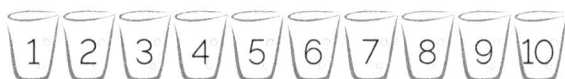

MY WINS I CELEBRATE TODAY ARE	TOMORROW I WILL IMPROVE ON

3 THINGS I AM THANKFUL FOR LAST 24 HOURS:

1. _____

2. _____

3. _____

THOUGHT DOWNLOAD

NOTES

MY WEEK OF AWESOMENESS!
Now that 6 month and monthly goals are done, we now can break down
our goals even further to make them even more achievable

REFLECTIONS OF LAST WEEK:

OBSTACLES I MAY FACE: _____

_____

SOLUTIONS: _____

_____

MY WEEK OF_____
Take 1-5 days this month to go through all your belongings and what you do not use regularly or have multiple of them is time to part with them. When parting with anything that is not actual trash, donate or sell these items.

TIME			

MY WEEK OF AWESOMENESS!

6 Month Goal	6 Month Goal
MONTH	MONTH
WEEK	WEEK
REWARD WHEN I REACH	REWARD WHEN I REACH

MY WEEK OF_____

What time do you want to wake up at, go to bed? How do you want your week to look like?

What events or meetings do you need to attend? Are you planning on having a day of shopping?

I WILL NOT BE DISRESPECTED BY ANYONE ESPECIALLY MYSELF!

AFFIRMATION OF THE DAY: _____

TODAY, I AM LOOKING FORWARD TO

GOALS #1

GOALS #2

HABITS I AM TRACKING	Y/N

THOUGHT DOWNLOAD

TODAY I AM CHOOSING TO FEEL:

C -

T -

F -
A -

R -

I WILL DRINK ___ GLASSES OF WATER TODAY: 1 2 3 4 5 6 7 8 9 10

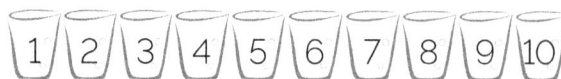

LOOKING BACK ON MY AMAZINGNESS

MY WINS I CELEBRATE TODAY ARE	TOMORROW I WILL IMPROVE ON

3 THINGS I AM THANKFUL FOR LAST 24 HOURS:

1. ______________________________

2. ______________________________

3. ______________________________

THOUGHT DOWNLOAD

NOTES

AFFIRMATION OF THE DAY: _____

TODAY, I AM LOOKING FORWARD TO

GOALS #1	GOALS #2	HABITS I AM TRACKING	Y/N

THOUGHT DOWNLOAD

TODAY I AM CHOOSING TO FEEL:

C -

T -

F -
A -

R -

I WILL DRINK ___ GLASSES OF WATER TODAY: 1 2 3 4 5 6 7 8 9 10

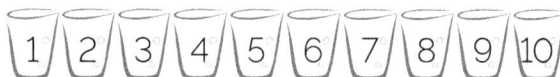

JENNIFER BULBROOK

LOOKING BACK ON MY AMAZINGNESS

MY WINS I CELEBRATE TODAY ARE	TOMORROW I WILL IMPROVE ON

3 THINGS I AM THANKFUL FOR LAST 24 HOURS:

1. ______________________________

2. ______________________________

3. ______________________________

THOUGHT DOWNLOAD

NOTES

AFFIRMATION OF THE DAY: _____

TODAY, I AM LOOKING FORWARD TO

GOALS #1

GOALS #2

HABITS I AM TRACKING	Y/N

THOUGHT DOWNLOAD

TODAY I AM CHOOSING TO FEEL:

C -

T -

F -
A -

R -

I WILL DRINK ___ GLASSES OF WATER TODAY: 1 2 3 4 5 6 7 8 9 10

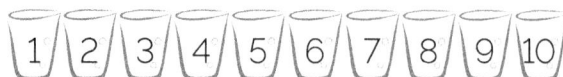

LOOKING BACK ON MY AMAZINGNESS

MY WINS I CELEBRATE TODAY ARE	TOMORROW I WILL IMPROVE ON

3 THINGS I AM THANKFUL FOR LAST 24 HOURS:

1. ______________________________

2. ______________________________

3. ______________________________

THOUGHT DOWNLOAD

NOTES

I WILL NOT PRETEND TO BE WHO I AM NOT!

AFFIRMATION OF THE DAY: _____

TODAY, I AM LOOKING FORWARD TO

GOALS #1	GOALS #2	HABITS I AM TRACKING	Y/N

THOUGHT DOWNLOAD

TODAY I AM CHOOSING TO FEEL:

C -

T -

F -
A -

R -

I WILL DRINK ___ GLASSES OF WATER TODAY: 1 2 3 4 5 6 7 8 9 10

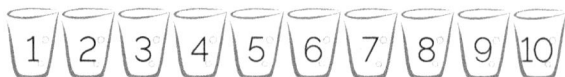

JENNIFER BULBROOK

LOOKING BACK ON MY AMAZINGNESS

MY WINS I CELEBRATE TODAY ARE	TOMORROW I WILL IMPROVE ON

3 THINGS I AM THANKFUL FOR LAST 24 HOURS:

1. ______________________________

2. ______________________________

3. ______________________________

THOUGHT DOWNLOAD

NOTES

AFFIRMATION OF THE DAY: _____

TODAY, I AM LOOKING FORWARD TO

GOALS #1	GOALS #2	HABITS I AM TRACKING	Y/N

THOUGHT DOWNLOAD

TODAY I AM CHOOSING TO FEEL:

C -

T -

F -
A -

R -

I WILL DRINK ___ GLASSES OF WATER TODAY: 1 2 3 4 5 6 7 8 9 10

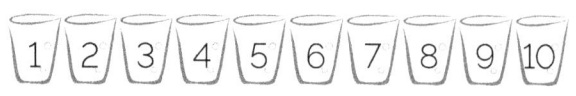

LOOKING BACK ON MY AMAZINGNESS

MY WINS I CELEBRATE TODAY ARE	TOMORROW I WILL IMPROVE ON

3 THINGS I AM THANKFUL FOR LAST 24 HOURS:

1. ______________________________

2. ______________________________

3. ______________________________

THOUGHT DOWNLOAD

NOTES

I WILL SHOW MYSELF RESPECT!

AFFIRMATION OF THE DAY: _____

TODAY, I AM LOOKING FORWARD TO

GOALS #1	GOALS #2	HABITS I AM TRACKING	Y/N

THOUGHT DOWNLOAD

TODAY I AM CHOOSING TO FEEL:

C -

T -

F -
A -

R -

I WILL DRINK ____ GLASSES OF WATER TODAY: 1 2 3 4 5 6 7 8 9 10

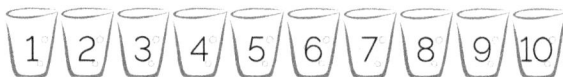

LOOKING BACK ON MY AMAZINGNESS

MY WINS I CELEBRATE TODAY ARE	TOMORROW I WILL IMPROVE ON

3 THINGS I AM THANKFUL FOR LAST 24 HOURS:

1. ____

2. ____

3. ____

THOUGHT DOWNLOAD

NOTES

AFFIRMATION OF THE DAY: _____

TODAY, I AM LOOKING FORWARD TO

GOALS #1

GOALS #2

HABITS I AM TRACKING	Y/N

THOUGHT DOWNLOAD

TODAY I AM CHOOSING TO FEEL:

C -

T -

F -
A -

R -

I WILL DRINK ___ GLASSES OF WATER TODAY: 1 2 3 4 5 6 7 8 9 10

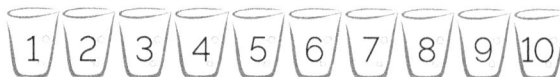

MY WINS I CELEBRATE TODAY ARE	TOMORROW I WILL IMPROVE ON

3 THINGS I AM THANKFUL FOR LAST 24 HOURS:

1. _____

2. _____

3. _____

THOUGHT DOWNLOAD

NOTES

MY WEEK OF AWESOMENESS!
Now that 6 month and monthly goals are done, we now can break down our goals even further to make them even more achievable

REFLECTIONS OF LAST WEEK:

OBSTACLES I MAY FACE: _____

_____

SOLUTIONS: _____

_____

MY WEEK OF_____
Take 1-5 days this month to go through all your belongings and what you do not use regularly or have multiple of them is time to part with them. When parting with anything that is not actual trash, donate or sell these items.

TIME			

MY WEEK OF AWESOMENESS!

6 Month Goal	6 Month Goal
MONTH	MONTH
WEEK	WEEK
REWARD WHEN I REACH	REWARD WHEN I REACH

MY WEEK OF_____

What time do you want to wake up at, go to bed? How do you want your week to look like?
What events or meetings do you need to attend? Are you planning on having a day of shopping?

AFFIRMATION OF THE DAY: _____

TODAY, I AM LOOKING FORWARD TO

GOALS #1	GOALS #2

HABITS I AM TRACKING	Y/N

THOUGHT DOWNLOAD

TODAY I AM CHOOSING TO FEEL:

C -

T -

F -
A -

R -

I WILL DRINK ___ GLASSES OF WATER TODAY: 1 2 3 4 5 6 7 8 9 10

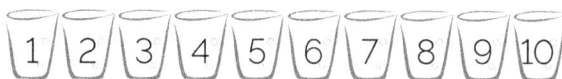

LOOKING BACK ON MY AMAZINGNESS

MY WINS I CELEBRATE TODAY ARE	TOMORROW I WILL IMPROVE ON

3 THINGS I AM THANKFUL FOR LAST 24 HOURS:

1. ______________________________

2. ______________________________

3. ______________________________

THOUGHT DOWNLOAD

NOTES

AFFIRMATION OF THE DAY: --

TODAY, I AM LOOKING FORWARD TO

GOALS #1	GOALS #2	HABITS I AM TRACKING	Y/N

THOUGHT DOWNLOAD

TODAY I AM CHOOSING TO FEEL:

C -

T -

F -

A -

R -

I WILL DRINK ___ GLASSES OF WATER TODAY: 1 2 3 4 5 6 7 8 9 10

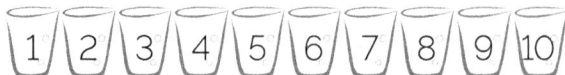

LOOKING BACK ON MY AMAZINGNESS

MY WINS I CELEBRATE TODAY ARE	TOMORROW I WILL IMPROVE ON

3 THINGS I AM THANKFUL FOR LAST 24 HOURS:

1. ____________________

2. ____________________

3. ____________________

THOUGHT DOWNLOAD

NOTES

AFFIRMATION OF THE DAY: _

TODAY, I AM LOOKING FORWARD TO

GOALS #1

GOALS #2

HABITS I AM TRACKING	Y/N

THOUGHT DOWNLOAD

TODAY I AM CHOOSING TO FEEL:

C -

T -

F -
A -

R -

I WILL DRINK ___ GLASSES OF WATER TODAY: 1 2 3 4 5 6 7 8 9 10

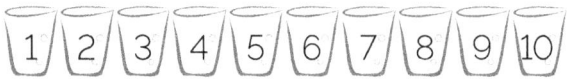

LOOKING BACK ON MY AMAZINGNESS

MY WINS I CELEBRATE TODAY ARE	TOMORROW I WILL IMPROVE ON

3 THINGS I AM THANKFUL FOR LAST 24 HOURS:

1. _____

2. _____

3. _____

THOUGHT DOWNLOAD

NOTES

AFFIRMATION OF THE DAY: --

TODAY, I AM LOOKING FORWARD TO

GOALS #1	GOALS #2

HABITS I AM TRACKING	Y/N

THOUGHT DOWNLOAD

TODAY I AM CHOOSING TO FEEL:

C -

T -

F -
A -

R -

I WILL DRINK ___ GLASSES OF WATER TODAY: 1 2 3 4 5 6 7 8 9 10

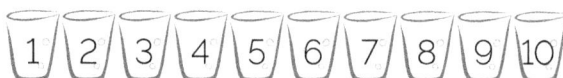

LOOKING BACK ON MY AMAZINGNESS

MY WINS I CELEBRATE TODAY ARE	TOMORROW I WILL IMPROVE ON

3 THINGS I AM THANKFUL FOR LAST 24 HOURS:

1. ____________________

2. ____________________

3. ____________________

THOUGHT DOWNLOAD

NOTES

AFFIRMATION OF THE DAY: _____

TODAY, I AM LOOKING FORWARD TO

GOALS #1	GOALS #2	HABITS I AM TRACKING	Y/N

THOUGHT DOWNLOAD

TODAY I AM CHOOSING TO FEEL:

C -

T -

F -
A -

R -

I WILL DRINK ___ GLASSES OF WATER TODAY: 1 2 3 4 5 6 7 8 9 10

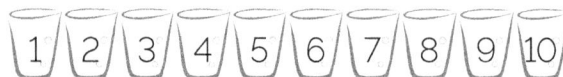

LOOKING BACK ON MY AMAZINGNESS

MY WINS I CELEBRATE TODAY ARE	TOMORROW I WILL IMPROVE ON

3 THINGS I AM THANKFUL FOR LAST 24 HOURS:

1. ______________________________

2. ______________________________

3. ______________________________

THOUGHT DOWNLOAD

NOTES

AFFIRMATION OF THE DAY: _____

TODAY, I AM LOOKING FORWARD TO

GOALS #1	GOALS #2	HABITS I AM TRACKING	Y/N

THOUGHT DOWNLOAD

TODAY I AM CHOOSING TO FEEL:

C -

T -

F -
A -

R -

I WILL DRINK ___ GLASSES OF WATER TODAY: 1 2 3 4 5 6 7 8 9 10

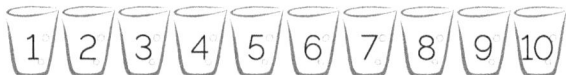

LOOKING BACK ON MY AMAZINGNESS

MY WINS I CELEBRATE TODAY ARE	TOMORROW I WILL IMPROVE ON

3 THINGS I AM THANKFUL FOR LAST 24 HOURS:

1. ______________________________

2. ______________________________

3. ______________________________

THOUGHT DOWNLOAD

NOTES

AFFIRMATION OF THE DAY: _

TODAY, I AM LOOKING FORWARD TO

GOALS #1	GOALS #2

HABITS I AM TRACKING	Y/N

THOUGHT DOWNLOAD

TODAY I AM CHOOSING TO FEEL:

C -

T -

F -
A -

R -

I WILL DRINK ___ GLASSES OF WATER TODAY: 1 2 3 4 5 6 7 8 9 10

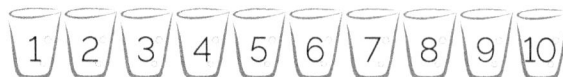

LOOKING BACK ON MY AMAZINGNESS

MY WINS I CELEBRATE TODAY ARE	TOMORROW I WILL IMPROVE ON

3 THINGS I AM THANKFUL FOR LAST 24 HOURS:

1. ______________________________

2. ______________________________

3. ______________________________

THOUGHT DOWNLOAD

NOTES

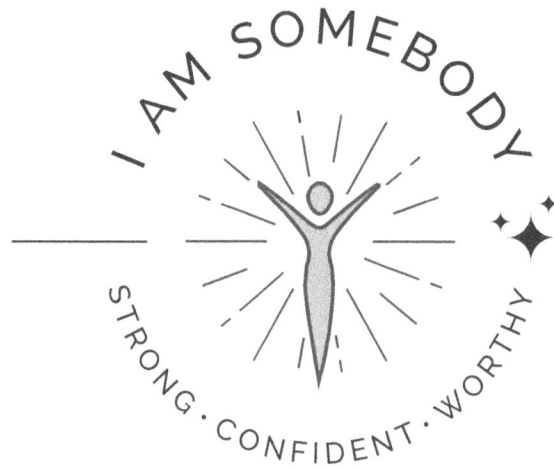

I AM SOMBODY

Transform Your Life Organizer™

Month Six

REJECTION

Rejection invites fear instead of confidence. Do not let your fears stand in the way of feeling worthy.Self-esteem and self-confidence are tied into our self-worth and to have a high sense of self-worth we must accept ourselves completely, the good, "the flaws", everything and that is what we will be working on over the next few weeks.

Are you a people pleaser? Do you want to please everyone? Do you fear just the thought of rejection?

In order not to feel or deal with rejection or the disapproval of others, you'll end up spending so much time doing nothing. That is what was happening to me; I was doing things that I had no interest in doing: eating things I did not even like, talking about things that I could frankly care less about, I was not voicing my opinions, needs or wants and why? Just so I would not have to deal with anyone else being disappointed or upset with me. Recently I made a commitment to myself that the only person I need to please is me. Yes, that is right, myself, not my boyfriend, not my family or friends, not even my kids. Now I am not saying that I am going to be selfish from this day forward and only do what I want but what I am saying is that I am not going to reject myself to protect myself from being rejected by others. I am taking responsibility for myself and for my circumstances as well as challenges. If I don't act and speak up for myself then how can I live a happy life? Being a people pleaser is giving all your power away to everyone but you. Who wants to do that?

Rejection will remain no matter what we do. We cannot and should not try to please everyone. No need to fret about it, take the time to embrace it because confidence comes from our willingness to experience the rejection others are willing to give. Do what you want, do what you love and are willing to accept. Rejection is not a big deal; it happens to everyone. If you really think about it anyways, rejection is what we make it, how we decide to feel about it.

Failure: Failure is always an option but guess what? The worst thing about failure is how we feel about it. Most people would say that there is nothing worse than failing but not me. I believe that what is worse than failing is not trying; that's quitting before the game even starts.

So many of us are afraid of failure that we dismiss it before even putting in an effort, and well frankly my friends, that is just sad. It took me years and years to finally say, hey, I am worthy enough to build my own Brand which is going to help millions of people and go through with it. Yes, I will make mistakes and yes there is a possibility that I may fail but I am going to do this because it is something I genuinely believe in. It has not been an easy process and there were many mistakes along the way but at one point I had said enough and just move forward. Why ? Because I Am Somebody!

I decided it was my time to shine and I will not give up on my dreams or myself. I am giving it my all. I can feel the achievements and successes in the pit of my stomach, I have such great excitement as I write this. There is no other option. Giving up is usually done in a rush and there is negative emotion associated with it. Acceptance is realizing there is nothing more you can do and that you've tried all that you know.

Knowing this, failure is going to happen, it is meant to happen, it is how we grow. Failure is just something not working out the way we hoped, how horrible is that? It is not really, not if we do not make it into a horrible thing. Did not happen the way you wanted, maybe there is a better thing that is going to happen or a better path for you. So, pick up your expectations, do not be afraid to fail, get out there and start failing because that is where your confidence comes in, from failing.

When we try new things and putt ourselves out there, we feel uncomfortable. That is when is when most people want to quit, tune out, and avoid what is going on. It is these exact moments that will either keep you exactly where you are if you are or create the strength within you that your next level requires if you choose to feel the discomfort and work through it.

The next tasks may require that you get out of your comfort zone. Let it be, feel it, work through it and you will automatically win!

HERE ARE 15 WAYS TO STOP YOURSELF FROM QUITTING

1. Understand what triggers you

2. Find the reason why you want to change

3. Hold yourself accountable to one human – YOU!

4. Be mindful of your thoughts

5. Swap a bad habit with a good one

6. Set reminders with post-its or on your phone

7. Prepare for mistakes

8. Let go of the All or Nothing mentality

9. Visualize it

10. Self care first and foremost

11. Reward yourself along the way

12. Believe in yourself

13. Know you are worth it

14. Find a support network

15. Remember … Say it with me… "I AM SOMEBODY

Here are a few key items that help me not only motivate me to keep going but they help me excel!

- Visualizing for 10-20 minutes a day. I focus on my future as if it is here and now in the present moment. This helps me remain committed to my dreams. I can feel the tingles in my stomach and the hairs stand up on my arms as if my website is already up and running with a million satisfied clients that I help. I can envision it and have the excitement and pride as if it is happening now and that is what helps me keep going.

- Stop making excuses whether it is lack of time, or holding onto the past or lack of self- confidence

- Think of the compound effect and how continuing to show up each day will add up. Achieving goals is not about an instant reward but about the process and growth that we experience. Write 1 page a day and in 365 days you will have a book. Take a snapshot of your typical day and time it by 365 days and then ask yourself if you would be satisfied?

Remember … Say it with me… "I AM SOMEBODY

"We think we fail and go backward. We only go back when we give up.
WHEN WE FAIL, WE ARE ACTUALLY MOVING FORWARD" Brooke Castillo

JENNIFER BULBROOK

Take full responsibility for everything that happens to you without giving your personal power away.

Ways to keep your power

- No complaining
- Accept responsibility for how you feel
- Do not hold grudges, practice forgiveness
- Do not waste time on unproductive thoughts.
- Move away from doubting and just do the doing part
- Avoid using "victim" language
- Establish healthy boundaries with yourself and others
- It is ok if not everyone likes you.
- Avoid any negative talk about yourself or others

Acknowledge that you have the personal power to change and influence the events and circumstances of your life.

PERSONAL BOUNDARIES

	NEVER	RARELY	SOMETIMES	OFTEN
I am having a difficult time saying no				
I have a difficult time asking for what I want or need				
I lack assertiveness				
I have a hard time making decisions				
I have a hard time knowing what I want				
I have a hard time knowing what I think and believe				
I do not like to disagree or have arguments				
I avoid conflict				
My happiness depends on other people				
Other people's opinions are more important than mine				
Other people know more than me				

NOT SURE WHERE TO BEGIN NEXT?

That is fine, just follow the next exercises and it will all come together!

Here are some key areas of your life. Examine which areas are the most important to you. Please give each of these areas a score of 1 to 10 (10 being the most important to you). You can use the same score more than once.

⚐	JOB/CAREER/EDUCATION	⚐	FINANCES
⚐	MENTAL HEALTH	⚐	PHYSICAL HEALTH
⚐	LEISURE TIME	⚐	HOME LIFE
⚐	RELATIONSHIPS – FAMILY/FRIENDS/ROMANTIC		

Look at your score. What are your top three important areas in your life, take a minute to write them below?

⚐

⚐

⚐

Ask yourself if there is anything you want to change or improve on in those areas? How satisfied are you with those areas in your life? Score each one from 1 to 10 (10 being the most satisfied) Are these areas serving you?

REMEMBER TO BE ENTERED INTO A DRAW, TAKE A SHORT VIDEO OF YOUR COMPLETED PLANNER, POST AND TAG @IAM_SOMEBODY_2 ON INSTAGRAM

MONTHLY GOALS

YOU ARE SO CLOSE, FINISH STRONG:

"The fact that someone else loves you doesn't rescue you from the project of loving yourself" Sahaj Kohli

6 MONTHS GOAL	MONTHLY GOAL
GOAL #1	
GOAL #2	

MONTH AT A GLANCE -

FNOW IS THE TIME TO SHINE

NOTES			

JENNIFER BULBROOK

BE REAL! BE YOU! THAT IS WHO WE ALL WANT TO SEE AND KNOW!

Every Sunday review & re-evaluate your goals. Identify obstacles that you faced, along with solutions.

		THROW YOUR SHOULDERS BACK AND WALK FASTER THAN THE AVERAGE PERSON!	Say it with me... I AM SOMEBODY

MY WEEK OF AWESOMENESS!
Now that 6 month and monthly goals are done, we now can break down
our goals even further to make them even more achievable

REFLECTIONS OF LAST WEEK:

OBSTACLES I MAY FACE: _____

_____

SOLUTIONS: _____

_____

MY WEEK OF_____
Take 1-5 days this month to go through all your belongings and what you do not use regularly or have multiple of them is time to part with them. When parting with anything that is not actual trash, donate or sell these items.

TIME			

MY WEEK OF AWESOMENESS!

6 Month Goal	6 Month Goal
MONTH	MONTH
WEEK	WEEK
REWARD WHEN I REACH	REWARD WHEN I REACH

MY WEEK OF _____

What time do you want to wake up at, go to bed? How do you want your week to look like?
What events or meetings do you need to attend? Are you planning on having a day of shopping?

AFFIRMATION OF THE DAY: _____

TODAY, I AM LOOKING FORWARD TO

GOALS #1	GOALS #2	HABITS I AM TRACKING	Y/N

THOUGHT DOWNLOAD

TODAY I AM CHOOSING TO FEEL:

C -

T -

F -
A -

R -

I WILL DRINK ___ GLASSES OF WATER TODAY: 1 2 3 4 5 6 7 8 9 10

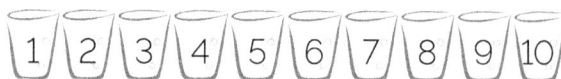

LOOKING BACK ON MY AMAZINGNESS

MY WINS I CELEBRATE TODAY ARE	TOMORROW I WILL IMPROVE ON

3 THINGS I AM THANKFUL FOR LAST 24 HOURS:

1. ______________________________

2. ______________________________

3. ______________________________

THOUGHT DOWNLOAD

NOTES

AFFIRMATION OF THE DAY: _____

TODAY, I AM LOOKING FORWARD TO

GOALS #1	GOALS #2

HABITS I AM TRACKING	Y/N

THOUGHT DOWNLOAD

TODAY I AM CHOOSING TO FEEL:

C -

T -

F -
A -

R -

I WILL DRINK ___ GLASSES OF WATER TODAY: 1 2 3 4 5 6 7 8 9 10

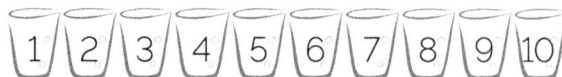

LOOKING BACK ON MY AMAZINGNESS

MY WINS I CELEBRATE TODAY ARE	TOMORROW I WILL IMPROVE ON

3 THINGS I AM THANKFUL FOR LAST 24 HOURS:

1. ______________________________

2. ______________________________

3. ______________________________

THOUGHT DOWNLOAD

NOTES

AFFIRMATION OF THE DAY: --

TODAY, I AM LOOKING FORWARD TO

GOALS #1	GOALS #2	HABITS I AM TRACKING	Y/N

THOUGHT DOWNLOAD

TODAY I AM CHOOSING TO FEEL:

C -

T -

F -
A -

R -

I WILL DRINK ___ GLASSES OF WATER TODAY: 1 2 3 4 5 6 7 8 9 10

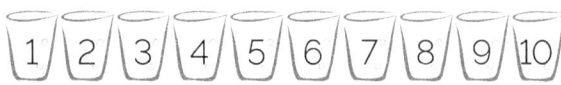

LOOKING BACK ON MY AMAZINGNESS

MY WINS I CELEBRATE TODAY ARE	TOMORROW I WILL IMPROVE ON

3 THINGS I AM THANKFUL FOR LAST 24 HOURS:

1. ______________________________

2. ______________________________

3. ______________________________

THOUGHT DOWNLOAD

NOTES

AFFIRMATION OF THE DAY: _____

TODAY, I AM LOOKING FORWARD TO

GOALS #1	GOALS #2

HABITS I AM TRACKING	Y/N

THOUGHT DOWNLOAD

TODAY I AM CHOOSING TO FEEL:

C -

T -

F -
A -

R -

I WILL DRINK ___ GLASSES OF WATER TODAY: 1 2 3 4 5 6 7 8 9 10

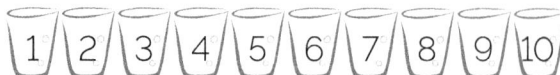

LOOKING BACK ON MY AMAZINGNESS

MY WINS I CELEBRATE TODAY ARE	TOMORROW I WILL IMPROVE ON

3 THINGS I AM THANKFUL FOR LAST 24 HOURS:

1. ____________________

2. ____________________

3. ____________________

THOUGHT DOWNLOAD

NOTES

AFFIRMATION OF THE DAY: _____

TODAY, I AM LOOKING FORWARD TO

GOALS #1	GOALS #2

HABITS I AM TRACKING	Y/N

THOUGHT DOWNLOAD

TODAY I AM CHOOSING TO FEEL:

C -

T -

F -
A -

R -

I WILL DRINK ___ GLASSES OF WATER TODAY: 1 2 3 4 5 6 7 8 9 10

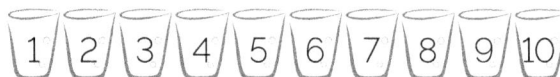

LOOKING BACK ON MY AMAZINGNESS

MY WINS I CELEBRATE TODAY ARE	TOMORROW I WILL IMPROVE ON

3 THINGS I AM THANKFUL FOR LAST 24 HOURS:

1. ______________________________

2. ______________________________

3. ______________________________

THOUGHT DOWNLOAD

NOTES

AFFIRMATION OF THE DAY: --

TODAY, I AM LOOKING FORWARD TO

GOALS #1	GOALS #2

HABITS I AM TRACKING	Y/N

THOUGHT DOWNLOAD

TODAY I AM CHOOSING TO FEEL:

C -

T -

F -
A -

R -

I WILL DRINK ___ GLASSES OF WATER TODAY: 1 2 3 4 5 6 7 8 9 10

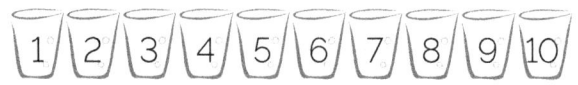

MY WINS I CELEBRATE TODAY ARE	TOMORROW I WILL IMPROVE ON

3 THINGS I AM THANKFUL FOR LAST 24 HOURS:

1. --

2. --

3. --

THOUGHT DOWNLOAD

NOTES

AFFIRMATION OF THE DAY: --

TODAY, I AM LOOKING FORWARD TO

GOALS #1	GOALS #2	HABITS I AM TRACKING	Y/N

THOUGHT DOWNLOAD

TODAY I AM CHOOSING TO FEEL:

C -

T -

F -
A -

R -

I WILL DRINK ___ GLASSES OF WATER TODAY: 1 2 3 4 5 6 7 8 9 10

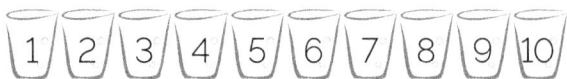

MY WINS I CELEBRATE TODAY ARE	TOMORROW I WILL IMPROVE ON

3 THINGS I AM THANKFUL FOR LAST 24 HOURS:

1. _____

2. _____

3. _____

THOUGHT DOWNLOAD

NOTES

MY WEEK OF AWESOMENESS!
Now that 6 month and monthly goals are done, we now can break down
our goals even further to make them even more achievable

REFLECTIONS OF LAST WEEK:

OBSTACLES I MAY FACE: _____

_____

SOLUTIONS: _____

_____

MY WEEK OF_____
Take 1-5 days this month to go through all your belongings and what you do not use regularly or have multiple of
them is time to part with them. When parting with anything that is not actual trash, donate or sell these items.

TIME			

JENNIFER BULBROOK

MY WEEK OF AWESOMENESS!

6 Month Goal	6 Month Goal
MONTH	MONTH
WEEK	WEEK
REWARD WHEN I REACH	REWARD WHEN I REACH

MY WEEK OF_____

What time do you want to wake up at, go to bed? How do you want your week to look like?

What events or meetings do you need to attend? Are you planning on having a day of shopping?

AFFIRMATION OF THE DAY: _____

TODAY, I AM LOOKING FORWARD TO

GOALS #1	GOALS #2	HABITS I AM TRACKING	Y/N

THOUGHT DOWNLOAD

TODAY I AM CHOOSING TO FEEL:

C -

T -

F -
A -

R -

I WILL DRINK ___ GLASSES OF WATER TODAY: 1 2 3 4 5 6 7 8 9 10

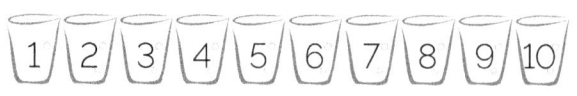

LOOKING BACK ON MY AMAZINGNESS

MY WINS I CELEBRATE TODAY ARE	TOMORROW I WILL IMPROVE ON

3 THINGS I AM THANKFUL FOR LAST 24 HOURS:

1. ______________________________

2. ______________________________

3. ______________________________

THOUGHT DOWNLOAD

NOTES

MANY PEOPLE LOVE AND ADMIRE ME!

AFFIRMATION OF THE DAY: _____

TODAY, I AM LOOKING FORWARD TO

GOALS #1	GOALS #2

HABITS I AM TRACKING	Y/N

THOUGHT DOWNLOAD

TODAY I AM CHOOSING TO FEEL:

C -

T -

F -
A -

R -

I WILL DRINK ___ GLASSES OF WATER TODAY: 1 2 3 4 5 6 7 8 9 10

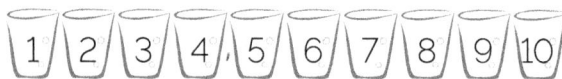

LOOKING BACK ON MY AMAZINGNESS

MY WINS I CELEBRATE TODAY ARE	TOMORROW I WILL IMPROVE ON

3 THINGS I AM THANKFUL FOR LAST 24 HOURS:

1. ______________________________

2. ______________________________

3. ______________________________

THOUGHT DOWNLOAD

NOTES

AFFIRMATION OF THE DAY: _____

TODAY, I AM LOOKING FORWARD TO

GOALS #1	GOALS #2

HABITS I AM TRACKING	Y/N

THOUGHT DOWNLOAD

TODAY I AM CHOOSING TO FEEL:

C -

T -

F -
A -

R -

I WILL DRINK ___ GLASSES OF WATER TODAY: 1 2 3 4 5 6 7 8 9 10

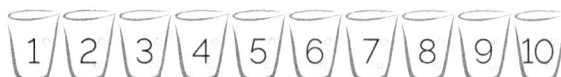

LOOKING BACK ON MY AMAZINGNESS

MY WINS I CELEBRATE TODAY ARE	TOMORROW I WILL IMPROVE ON

3 THINGS I AM THANKFUL FOR LAST 24 HOURS:

1. ________________

2. ________________

3. ________________

THOUGHT DOWNLOAD

NOTES

I AM HAPPY!

AFFIRMATION OF THE DAY: _____

TODAY, I AM LOOKING FORWARD TO

GOALS #1	GOALS #2	HABITS I AM TRACKING	Y/N

THOUGHT DOWNLOAD

TODAY I AM CHOOSING TO FEEL:

C -

T -

F -
A -

R -

I WILL DRINK ___ GLASSES OF WATER TODAY: 1 2 3 4 5 6 7 8 9 10

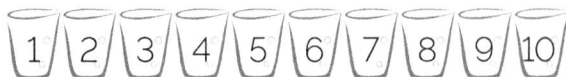

JENNIFER BULBROOK

LOOKING BACK ON MY AMAZINGNESS

MY WINS I CELEBRATE TODAY ARE	TOMORROW I WILL IMPROVE ON

3 THINGS I AM THANKFUL FOR LAST 24 HOURS:

1. ______________________________

2. ______________________________

3. ______________________________

THOUGHT DOWNLOAD

NOTES

AFFIRMATION OF THE DAY: _____

TODAY, I AM LOOKING FORWARD TO

GOALS #1	GOALS #2	HABITS I AM TRACKING	Y/N

THOUGHT DOWNLOAD

TODAY I AM CHOOSING TO FEEL:

C -

T -

F -
A -

R -

I WILL DRINK ___ GLASSES OF WATER TODAY: 1 2 3 4 5 6 7 8 9 10

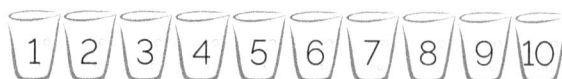

LOOKING BACK ON MY AMAZINGNESS

MY WINS I CELEBRATE TODAY ARE	TOMORROW I WILL IMPROVE ON

3 THINGS I AM THANKFUL FOR LAST 24 HOURS:

1. ____

2. ____

3. ____

THOUGHT DOWNLOAD

NOTES

AFFIRMATION OF THE DAY: --

TODAY, I AM LOOKING FORWARD TO

GOALS #1	GOALS #2	HABITS I AM TRACKING	Y/N

THOUGHT DOWNLOAD

TODAY I AM CHOOSING TO FEEL:

C -

T -

F -
A -

R -

I WILL DRINK ____ GLASSES OF WATER TODAY: 1 2 3 4 5 6 7 8 9 10

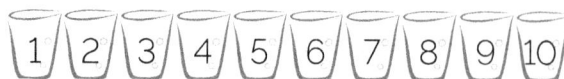

LOOKING BACK ON MY AMAZINGNESS

MY WINS I CELEBRATE TODAY ARE	TOMORROW I WILL IMPROVE ON

3 THINGS I AM THANKFUL FOR LAST 24 HOURS:

1. ______________________________

2. ______________________________

3. ______________________________

THOUGHT DOWNLOAD

NOTES

AFFIRMATION OF THE DAY: _____

TODAY, I AM LOOKING FORWARD TO

GOALS #1	GOALS #2	HABITS I AM TRACKING	Y/N

THOUGHT DOWNLOAD

TODAY I AM CHOOSING TO FEEL:

C -

T -

F -
A -

R -

I WILL DRINK ___ GLASSES OF WATER TODAY: 1 2 3 4 5 6 7 8 9 10

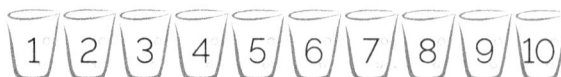

LOOKING BACK ON MY AMAZINGNESS

MY WINS I CELEBRATE TODAY ARE	TOMORROW I WILL IMPROVE ON

3 THINGS I AM THANKFUL FOR LAST 24 HOURS:

1. _____

2. _____

3. _____

THOUGHT DOWNLOAD

NOTES

MY WEEK OF AWESOMENESS!
Now that 6 month and monthly goals are done, we now can break down
our goals even further to make them even more achievable

REFLECTIONS OF LAST WEEK:

OBSTACLES I MAY FACE: _____

_____

SOLUTIONS: _____

_____

MY WEEK OF_____
Take 1-5 days this month to go through all your belongings and what you do not use regularly or have multiple of
them is time to part with them. When parting with anything that is not actual trash, donate or sell these items.

TIME			

JENNIFER BULBROOK

MY WEEK OF AWESOMENESS!

6 Month Goal	6 Month Goal
MONTH	MONTH
WEEK	WEEK
REWARD WHEN I REACH	REWARD WHEN I REACH

MY WEEK OF_____

What time do you want to wake up at, go to bed? How do you want your week to look like?
What events or meetings do you need to attend? Are you planning on having a day of shopping?

AFFIRMATION OF THE DAY: _____

TODAY, I AM LOOKING FORWARD TO

GOALS #1	GOALS #2

HABITS I AM TRACKING	Y/N

THOUGHT DOWNLOAD

TODAY I AM CHOOSING TO FEEL:

C -

T -

F -
A -

R -

I WILL DRINK ____ GLASSES OF WATER TODAY: 1 2 3 4 5 6 7 8 9 10

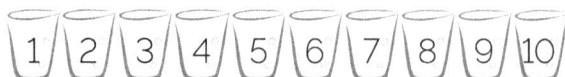

LOOKING BACK ON MY AMAZINGNESS

MY WINS I CELEBRATE TODAY ARE	TOMORROW I WILL IMPROVE ON

3 THINGS I AM THANKFUL FOR LAST 24 HOURS:

1. ______________________________

2. ______________________________

3. ______________________________

THOUGHT DOWNLOAD

NOTES

AFFIRMATION OF THE DAY: _____

TODAY, I AM LOOKING FORWARD TO

GOALS #1	GOALS #2	HABITS I AM TRACKING	Y/N

THOUGHT DOWNLOAD

TODAY I AM CHOOSING TO FEEL:

C -

T -

F -
A -

R -

I WILL DRINK ___ GLASSES OF WATER TODAY: 1 2 3 4 5 6 7 8 9 10

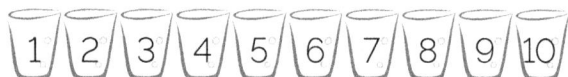

LOOKING BACK ON MY AMAZINGNESS

MY WINS I CELEBRATE TODAY ARE	TOMORROW I WILL IMPROVE ON

3 THINGS I AM THANKFUL FOR LAST 24 HOURS:

1. ____________________
2. ____________________
3. ____________________

THOUGHT DOWNLOAD

NOTES

I KNOW I HAVE PEOPLE WHO NEED ME EVEN WHEN I CAN'T SEE MY WORTH!

AFFIRMATION OF THE DAY: _____

TODAY, I AM LOOKING FORWARD TO

GOALS #1

GOALS #2

HABITS I AM TRACKING	Y/N

THOUGHT DOWNLOAD

TODAY I AM CHOOSING TO FEEL:

C -

T -

F -
A -

R -

I WILL DRINK ___ GLASSES OF WATER TODAY: 1 2 3 4 5 6 7 8 9 10

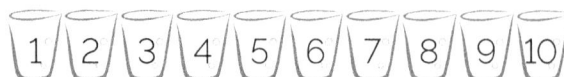

JENNIFER BULBROOK

LOOKING BACK ON MY AMAZINGNESS

MY WINS I CELEBRATE TODAY ARE	TOMORROW I WILL IMPROVE ON

3 THINGS I AM THANKFUL FOR LAST 24 HOURS:

1. ______________________________

2. ______________________________

3. ______________________________

THOUGHT DOWNLOAD

NOTES

AFFIRMATION OF THE DAY: _____

TODAY, I AM LOOKING FORWARD TO

GOALS #1	GOALS #2	HABITS I AM TRACKING	Y/N

THOUGHT DOWNLOAD

TODAY I AM CHOOSING TO FEEL:

C -

T -

F -
A -

R -

I WILL DRINK ____ GLASSES OF WATER TODAY: 1 2 3 4 5 6 7 8 9 10

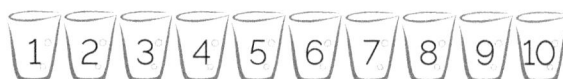

LOOKING BACK ON MY AMAZINGNESS

MY WINS I CELEBRATE TODAY ARE	TOMORROW I WILL IMPROVE ON

3 THINGS I AM THANKFUL FOR LAST 24 HOURS:

1. ______________________________

2. ______________________________

3. ______________________________

THOUGHT DOWNLOAD

NOTES

AFFIRMATION OF THE DAY: _____

TODAY, I AM LOOKING FORWARD TO

GOALS #1	GOALS #2

HABITS I AM TRACKING	Y/N

THOUGHT DOWNLOAD

TODAY I AM CHOOSING TO FEEL:

C -

T -

F -
A -

R -

I WILL DRINK ___ GLASSES OF WATER TODAY: 1 2 3 4 5 6 7 8 9 10

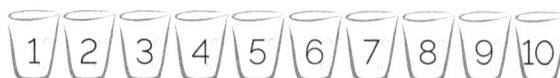

LOOKING BACK ON MY AMAZINGNESS

MY WINS I CELEBRATE TODAY ARE	TOMORROW I WILL IMPROVE ON

3 THINGS I AM THANKFUL FOR LAST 24 HOURS:

1. _____

2. _____

3. _____

THOUGHT DOWNLOAD

NOTES

AFFIRMATION OF THE DAY: ---

TODAY, I AM LOOKING FORWARD TO

GOALS #1	GOALS #2	HABITS I AM TRACKING	Y/N

THOUGHT DOWNLOAD

TODAY I AM CHOOSING TO FEEL:

C -

T -

F -
A -

R -

I WILL DRINK ___ GLASSES OF WATER TODAY: 1 2 3 4 5 6 7 8 9 10

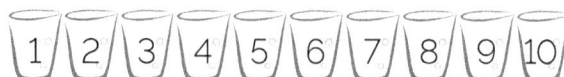

LOOKING BACK ON MY AMAZINGNESS

MY WINS I CELEBRATE TODAY ARE	TOMORROW I WILL IMPROVE ON

3 THINGS I AM THANKFUL FOR LAST 24 HOURS:

1. ____________________

2. ____________________

3. ____________________

THOUGHT DOWNLOAD

NOTES

AFFIRMATION OF THE DAY: _____

TODAY, I AM LOOKING FORWARD TO

GOALS #1	GOALS #2	HABITS I AM TRACKING	Y/N

THOUGHT DOWNLOAD

TODAY I AM CHOOSING TO FEEL:

C -

T -

F -
A -

R -

I WILL DRINK ___ GLASSES OF WATER TODAY: 1 2 3 4 5 6 7 8 9 10

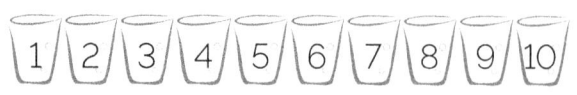

LOOKING BACK ON MY AMAZINGNESS

MY WINS I CELEBRATE TODAY ARE	TOMORROW I WILL IMPROVE ON

3 THINGS I AM THANKFUL FOR LAST 24 HOURS:

1. _____

2. _____

3. _____

THOUGHT DOWNLOAD

NOTES

MY WEEK OF AWESOMENESS!
Now that 6 month and monthly goals are done, we now can break down
our goals even further to make them even more achievable

REFLECTIONS OF LAST WEEK:

OBSTACLES I MAY FACE: _____

_____

SOLUTIONS: _____

_____

MY WEEK OF_____
Take 1-5 days this month to go through all your belongings and what you do not use regularly or have multiple of them is time to part with them. When parting with anything that is not actual trash, donate or sell these items.

TIME			

MY WEEK OF AWESOMENESS!

6 Month Goal	6 Month Goal
MONTH	MONTH
WEEK	WEEK
REWARD WHEN I REACH	REWARD WHEN I REACH

MY WEEK OF_____

What time do you want to wake up at, go to bed? How do you want your week to look like?
What events or meetings do you need to attend? Are you planning on having a day of shopping?

AFFIRMATION OF THE DAY: _____

TODAY, I AM LOOKING FORWARD TO

GOALS #1

GOALS #2

HABITS I AM TRACKING	Y/N

THOUGHT DOWNLOAD

TODAY I AM CHOOSING TO FEEL:

C -

T -

F -
A -

R -

I WILL DRINK ___ GLASSES OF WATER TODAY: 1 2 3 4 5 6 7 8 9 10

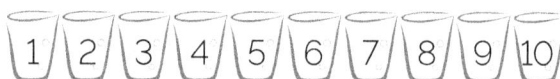

LOOKING BACK ON MY AMAZINGNESS

MY WINS I CELEBRATE TODAY ARE	TOMORROW I WILL IMPROVE ON

3 THINGS I AM THANKFUL FOR LAST 24 HOURS:

1. ______________________________

2. ______________________________

3. ______________________________

THOUGHT DOWNLOAD

NOTES

AFFIRMATION OF THE DAY: --

TODAY, I AM LOOKING FORWARD TO

GOALS #1	GOALS #2

HABITS I AM TRACKING	Y/N

THOUGHT DOWNLOAD

TODAY I AM CHOOSING TO FEEL:

C -

T -

F -
A -

R -

I WILL DRINK ___ GLASSES OF WATER TODAY: 1 2 3 4 5 6 7 8 9 10

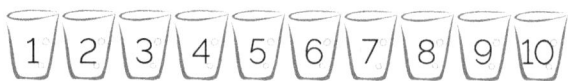

JENNIFER BULBROOK

LOOKING BACK ON MY AMAZINGNESS

MY WINS I CELEBRATE TODAY ARE	TOMORROW I WILL IMPROVE ON

3 THINGS I AM THANKFUL FOR LAST 24 HOURS:

1. ______________________________

2. ______________________________

3. ______________________________

THOUGHT DOWNLOAD

NOTES

I WILL NOT JUDGE MY FEELINGS!

AFFIRMATION OF THE DAY: _____

TODAY, I AM LOOKING FORWARD TO

GOALS #1	GOALS #2

HABITS I AM TRACKING	Y/N

THOUGHT DOWNLOAD

TODAY I AM CHOOSING TO FEEL:

C -

T -

F -
A -

R -

I WILL DRINK ___ GLASSES OF WATER TODAY: 1 2 3 4 5 6 7 8 9 10

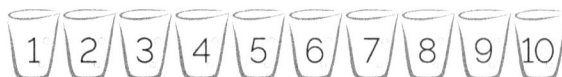

JENNIFER BULBROOK

LOOKING BACK ON MY AMAZINGNESS

MY WINS I CELEBRATE TODAY ARE	TOMORROW I WILL IMPROVE ON

3 THINGS I AM THANKFUL FOR LAST 24 HOURS:

1. ______________________________

2. ______________________________

3. ______________________________

THOUGHT DOWNLOAD

NOTES

AFFIRMATION OF THE DAY: _____

TODAY, I AM LOOKING FORWARD TO

GOALS #1	GOALS #2	HABITS I AM TRACKING	Y/N

THOUGHT DOWNLOAD

TODAY I AM CHOOSING TO FEEL:

C -

T -

F -
A -

R -

I WILL DRINK ___ GLASSES OF WATER TODAY: 1 2 3 4 5 6 7 8 9 10

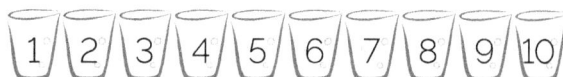

LOOKING BACK ON MY AMAZINGNESS

MY WINS I CELEBRATE TODAY ARE	TOMORROW I WILL IMPROVE ON

3 THINGS I AM THANKFUL FOR LAST 24 HOURS:

1. ____________________

2. ____________________

3. ____________________

THOUGHT DOWNLOAD

NOTES

AFFIRMATION OF THE DAY: _____

TODAY, I AM LOOKING FORWARD TO

GOALS #1	GOALS #2	HABITS I AM TRACKING	Y/N

THOUGHT DOWNLOAD

TODAY I AM CHOOSING TO FEEL:

C -

T -

F -
A -

R -

I WILL DRINK ____ GLASSES OF WATER TODAY: 1 2 3 4 5 6 7 8 9 10

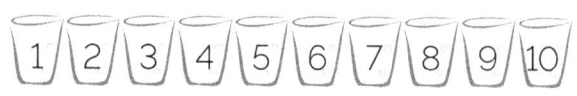

JENNIFER BULBROOK

LOOKING BACK ON MY AMAZINGNESS

MY WINS I CELEBRATE TODAY ARE	TOMORROW I WILL IMPROVE ON

3 THINGS I AM THANKFUL FOR LAST 24 HOURS:

1. ____________________

2. ____________________

3. ____________________

THOUGHT DOWNLOAD

NOTES

AFFIRMATION OF THE DAY: _____

TODAY, I AM LOOKING FORWARD TO

GOALS #1	GOALS #2	HABITS I AM TRACKING	Y/N

THOUGHT DOWNLOAD

TODAY I AM CHOOSING TO FEEL:

C -

T -

F -
A -

R -

I WILL DRINK ___ GLASSES OF WATER TODAY: 1 2 3 4 5 6 7 8 9 10

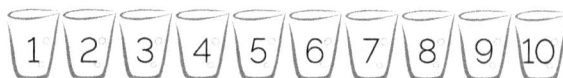

LOOKING BACK ON MY AMAZINGNESS

MY WINS I CELEBRATE TODAY ARE	TOMORROW I WILL IMPROVE ON

3 THINGS I AM THANKFUL FOR LAST 24 HOURS:

1. ____________________

2. ____________________

3. ____________________

THOUGHT DOWNLOAD

NOTES

AFFIRMATION OF THE DAY: _____

TODAY, I AM LOOKING FORWARD TO

GOALS #1	GOALS #2	HABITS I AM TRACKING	Y/N

THOUGHT DOWNLOAD

TODAY I AM CHOOSING TO FEEL:

C -

T -

F -
A -

R -

I WILL DRINK ___ GLASSES OF WATER TODAY: 1 2 3 4 5 6 7 8 9 10

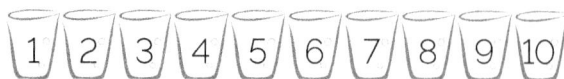

MY WINS I CELEBRATE TODAY ARE	TOMORROW I WILL IMPROVE ON

3 THINGS I AM THANKFUL FOR LAST 24 HOURS:

1. _____

2. _____

3. _____

THOUGHT DOWNLOAD

NOTES

MY WEEK OF AWESOMENESS!
Now that 6 month and monthly goals are done, we now can break down
our goals even further to make them even more achievable

REFLECTIONS OF LAST WEEK:

OBSTACLES I MAY FACE: _____

_____

SOLUTIONS: _____

_____

MY WEEK OF _____
Take 1-5 days this month to go through all your belongings and what you do not use regularly or have multiple of
them is time to part with them. When parting with anything that is not actual trash, donate or sell these items.

TIME			

MY WEEK OF AWESOMENESS!

6 Month Goal	6 Month Goal
MONTH	MONTH
WEEK	WEEK
REWARD WHEN I REACH	REWARD WHEN I REACH

MY WEEK OF_____

What time do you want to wake up at, go to bed? How do you want your week to look like?

What events or meetings do you need to attend? Are you planning on having a day of shopping?

AFFIRMATION OF THE DAY: _____

TODAY, I AM LOOKING FORWARD TO

GOALS #1	GOALS #2	HABITS I AM TRACKING	Y/N

THOUGHT DOWNLOAD

TODAY I AM CHOOSING TO FEEL:

C -

T -

F -
A -

R -

I WILL DRINK ___ GLASSES OF WATER TODAY: 1 2 3 4 5 6 7 8 9 10

LOOKING BACK ON MY AMAZINGNESS

MY WINS I CELEBRATE TODAY ARE	TOMORROW I WILL IMPROVE ON

3 THINGS I AM THANKFUL FOR LAST 24 HOURS:

1. ________________

2. ________________

3. ________________

THOUGHT DOWNLOAD

NOTES

AFFIRMATION OF THE DAY: _____

TODAY, I AM LOOKING FORWARD TO

GOALS #1	GOALS #2	HABITS I AM TRACKING	Y/N

THOUGHT DOWNLOAD

TODAY I AM CHOOSING TO FEEL:

C -

T -

F -
A -

R -

I WILL DRINK ___ GLASSES OF WATER TODAY: 1 2 3 4 5 6 7 8 9 10

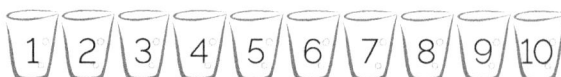

JENNIFER BULBROOK

LOOKING BACK ON MY AMAZINGNESS

MY WINS I CELEBRATE TODAY ARE	TOMORROW I WILL IMPROVE ON

3 THINGS I AM THANKFUL FOR LAST 24 HOURS:

1. ______________________________

2. ______________________________

3. ______________________________

THOUGHT DOWNLOAD

NOTES

AFFIRMATION OF THE DAY: _____

TODAY, I AM LOOKING FORWARD TO

GOALS #1	GOALS #2	HABITS I AM TRACKING	Y/N

THOUGHT DOWNLOAD

TODAY I AM CHOOSING TO FEEL:

C -

T -

F -
A -

R -

I WILL DRINK ___ GLASSES OF WATER TODAY: 1 2 3 4 5 6 7 8 9 10

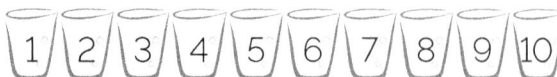

JENNIFER BULBROOK

LOOKING BACK ON MY AMAZINGNESS

MY WINS I CELEBRATE TODAY ARE	TOMORROW I WILL IMPROVE ON

3 THINGS I AM THANKFUL FOR LAST 24 HOURS:

1. ______________________________

2. ______________________________

3. ______________________________

THOUGHT DOWNLOAD

NOTES

AFFIRMATION OF THE DAY: _____

TODAY, I AM LOOKING FORWARD TO

GOALS #1	GOALS #2	HABITS I AM TRACKING	Y/N

THOUGHT DOWNLOAD

TODAY I AM CHOOSING TO FEEL:

C -

T -

F -
A -

R -

I WILL DRINK ____ GLASSES OF WATER TODAY: 1 2 3 4 5 6 7 8 9 10

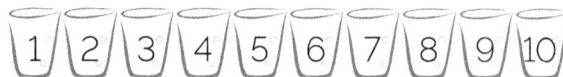

LOOKING BACK ON MY AMAZINGNESS

MY WINS I CELEBRATE TODAY ARE	TOMORROW I WILL IMPROVE ON

3 THINGS I AM THANKFUL FOR LAST 24 HOURS:

1. ______________________________

2. ______________________________

3. ______________________________

THOUGHT DOWNLOAD

NOTES

I AM VALUED BY MY FRIENDS AND FAMILY!

AFFIRMATION OF THE DAY: _____

TODAY, I AM LOOKING FORWARD TO

GOALS #1	GOALS #2

HABITS I AM TRACKING	Y/N

THOUGHT DOWNLOAD

TODAY I AM CHOOSING TO FEEL:

C -

T -

F -
A -

R -

I WILL DRINK ___ GLASSES OF WATER TODAY: 1 2 3 4 5 6 7 8 9 10

JENNIFER BULBROOK

LOOKING BACK ON MY AMAZINGNESS

MY WINS I CELEBRATE TODAY ARE	TOMORROW I WILL IMPROVE ON

3 THINGS I AM THANKFUL FOR LAST 24 HOURS:

1. ____________________

2. ____________________

3. ____________________

THOUGHT DOWNLOAD

NOTES

I WILL NOT LET ANYTHING GET IN THE WAY OF MY HAPPINESS!

AFFIRMATION OF THE DAY: _____

TODAY, I AM LOOKING FORWARD TO

GOALS #1	GOALS #2

HABITS I AM TRACKING	Y/N

THOUGHT DOWNLOAD

TODAY I AM CHOOSING TO FEEL:

C -

T -

F -
A -

R -

I WILL DRINK ___ GLASSES OF WATER TODAY: 1 2 3 4 5 6 7 8 9 10

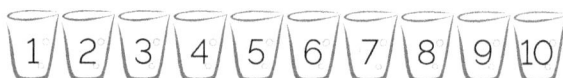

LOOKING BACK ON MY AMAZINGNESS

MY WINS I CELEBRATE TODAY ARE	TOMORROW I WILL IMPROVE ON

3 THINGS I AM THANKFUL FOR LAST 24 HOURS:

1. ______________________________

2. ______________________________

3. ______________________________

THOUGHT DOWNLOAD

NOTES

AFFIRMATION OF THE DAY: _____

TODAY, I AM LOOKING FORWARD TO

GOALS #1	GOALS #2	HABITS I AM TRACKING	Y/N

THOUGHT DOWNLOAD

TODAY I AM CHOOSING TO FEEL:

C -

T -

F -
A -

R -

I WILL DRINK ____ GLASSES OF WATER TODAY: 1 2 3 4 5 6 7 8 9 10

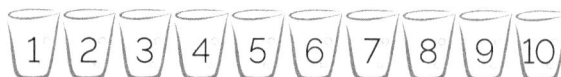

LOOKING BACK ON MY AMAZINGNESS

MY WINS I CELEBRATE TODAY ARE	TOMORROW I WILL IMPROVE ON

3 THINGS I AM THANKFUL FOR LAST 24 HOURS:

1. --

2. --

3. --

THOUGHT DOWNLOAD

NOTES

IT IS TO LOOK AT OUR LIVES AND DECIDE ON OUR NEXT STEPS!

Now it is time to begin to explore what you would like to focus on next. Where are you now and what do you want to create in your life? You may want to continue to work on your Self-Worth and go more in depth with respect to the tools that will transform your life and therefore want to invest in the 2nd edition of the Transform Your Life Organizer ™.

Visit http://www.IAMSOMEBODY2.CA at the various planners we offer.

- Feeling down, depressed?

- Lack of motivation?

- Experiencing anxiety and/or panic attacks?

- Are you in a rut that you just cannot seem to get out of?

- Tired of feeling uncomfortable?

- Feel as though your feelings are not always rational?

- Irritable and worrying too much?

- Looking for POSITIVE support?

- Then check out our organizers geared towards Depression or anxiety

- Drinking more than you would like?

- Popping an extra pill or 2 a day?

- Seems to have MOFO where you cannot be missing out on any of the fun?

- Do you do any type of hard drugs but not want to be?

- If you say yes to any of these questions, please know that I got you and so does our addiction organizer

- Having difficulty getting over an ex?

- I have an organizer just for you … Huh? What Ex?

ASK: Take the bull by the horns and do what you always wanted to do (but have been afraid of failing). Make a list of things you want to do, something that is important to you or something that you have been dying to do or learn. You can start small like learning to play the drums or the proper gardening techniques. Once you have a few ideas, I want you to decide which one you will actively work towards. Then plan the next steps and what needs to happen to achieve it. Then it is time to execute. Make sure you show up and you are prepared.

OUR SUCCESS STORIES - As human being, we are much better at remembering what went wrong and how we failed than our successes. Sometimes it is difficult to grasp the role you have had in your own or the success of others. It is therefore useful to keep track of your wins and your success stories. Whether you are keeping a digital or handwritten copy, complete the following to record all that has gone well, and then review regularly or before a future challenge:

SITUATION	DESCRIPTION
What was the situation?	
What was my involvement?	
What challenges did I face?	
What did I achieve?	
How did I feel?	

SITUATION	DESCRIPTION
What was the situation?	
What was my involvement?	
What challenges did I face?	
What did I achieve?	
How did I feel?	

SITUATION	DESCRIPTION
What was the situation?	
What was my involvement?	
What challenges did I face?	
What did I achieve?	
How did I feel?	

DEDICATION

This book is dedicated to my kids.

Through all the struggles you encounter please
always remember you are worthy,

You Are Somebody

Love Mom

A SPECIAL THANKYOU

for the resources which have been helping me throughout my journey.

www.thegoalchaser.com

www.neocody.medium.com

The Life Coach School Podcast

www.positivepsychology.com

www.merriam-webster.com/dictionary

www.proctorgallagherinstitute.com/

www.mayoclinic.org/diseases-conditions/depression/symptoms-causes/syc-20356007

www.happier.com

www.skillsyouneed.com

www.Dr. Christina Hibbert.com

How To Accept Yourself Fully: A Guide To Self-Acceptance

www.myamericannurse.com)

www.newsweeks.com/Humans Have More than 6,000 Thoughts per Day, Psychologists Discover (newsweek.com)

www.healthyplace.com

Rise Up by Moira Kucaba

I am Jennifer Bulbrook, the Founder and Owner of the new Canadian Brand, I Am Somebody and I will be your person to help you to your brand-new life which is waiting for you within these pages. My hope is to be able to not only inspire you but to teach you the tools and skills you need to fulfill your dreams and to stand proud as you scream, I Am Somebody

I was born and raised in Hamilton, Ontario, the middle child of a loving family. I have a background in Child and Youth Work as well as Law. I am currently enrolled in The Life Coach School while building this Canadian Brand to help give people the tools to have the best life they possibly canHere are some key areas of your life. Examine which areas are the most important to you. Please give each of these areas a score of 1 to 10 (10 being the most important to you). You can use the same score more than once.

I have a history with mental health. I spent most of my 9th grade year in the psychiatric ward for depression, self harm, and suicide attempts. At the age of 15 I turned to drugs, anything I could get my hands on. While addicted to drugs and partying every day, at the age of 17, I became pregnant. I was so excited, filled with joy as I was going to have the baby, I always grew up wanting to love me and for me to love him/her. Unfortunately, things did not work out as perfectly as this was when my addiction to alcohol began.

I have been working on these Self Transformation Planners, which are unlike any ordinary planner you have ever had or seen before; I have specifically designed each of these to contain the tools you need to change your life and to feel true happiness and to succeed in all that you do. Our Transformation Planners will feature self-development strategies, and each will be specifically geared towards topics such as self worth, depression, anxiety etc.

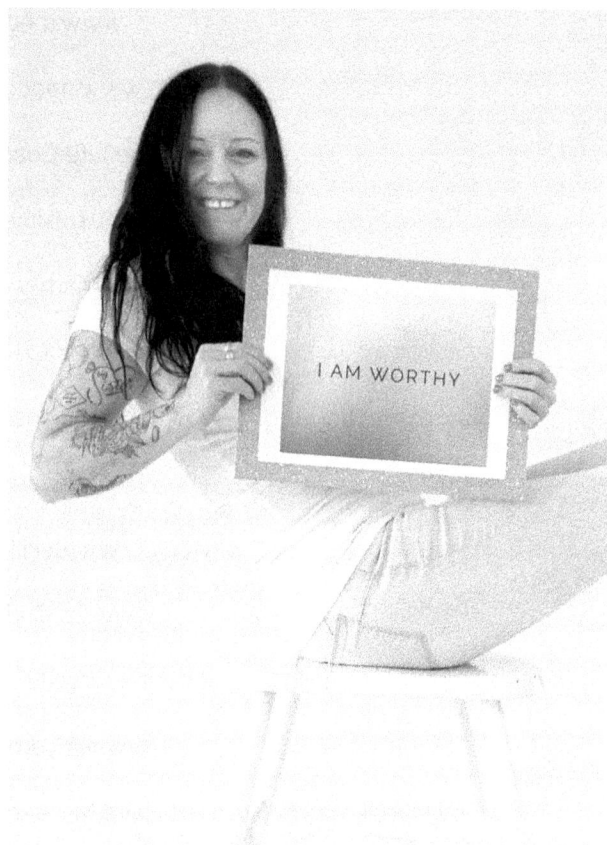

I am here to serve you in any way I can whether it be talking through your issues with me 1:1, starting to use my amazing and specifically designed planners, joining our incredible VIP community, or moving with me.

Whether you are suffering from addiction issues, mental health issues, want to focus on your weight or having a hard time getting over an ex, the I am Somebody community is here for you.

Because You Are Somebody And You Are Worth It